Get Buffed! ™ II

Ian King's Guide to getting BIGGER, STRONGER & LEANER!

King Sports Publishing
www.getbuffed.net
Email : info@getbuffed.net
Ph +1-775-327-4550 Fax +1-240-465-4873
1135 Terminal Way, Suite 209, Reno NV 89502, USA

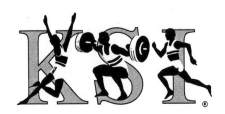

Published by:
King Sports Publishing
King Sports International
www.getbuffed.net
info@getbuffed.net
Ph +1-775-327-4550 Fax +1-240-465-4873
1135 Terminal Way, Suite 209, Reno NV 89502, USA

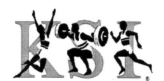

ISBN 1-920685-05-7
Title: Get Buffed! II Get More Buffed!
Edition: 1st
Author/Contributor: King, Ian
Date of Publication: Nov 2002   Price: $ 39.95 USD / $69.95 AUD
Format: PB   Size:295x210   No .of Pages: 317
Publisher: King Sports International

Disclaimer

This book is designed to provide information in regard to the subject matter covered. The purpose of this book is to educate. The author and publisher shall have neither liability nor responsibility to any person or entity with respect to any of the information contained in this book. It is recommend that you seek independent medical and training specialist advice before proceeding with any training method.

Acknowledgements

I want to say 'thanks' to all those who supported the original Get Buffed!™ book, both before and after it's release. Your support has made the original Get Buffed! ™ our best selling book, and given us the confidence to ahead and produce this book, the sequel to the original book.

From that original book, we have gone on to create a totally new range, appropriately titled the Get Buffed! ™ range! Videos, training diaries, and now this – a sequel to the original book!

To those who have placed their trust our Get Buffed! ™ range – a huge thank you from us! Your belief and support has ensured that what began with a single book has grown into a complete range.

Enjoy this sequel edition! May it take allow you to 'Get More Buffed'! Now go and Get Buffed!™

Ian King

Table of Contents

Foreword

Setting the scene

When I wrote the original *Get Buffed!*™ book in 1999, I introduced a number of concepts to the marketplace that were not conventional. I was aware of this, and I was aware that if I introduced too many of these lesser-known training concepts in this book, I ran the risk of being totally dismissed as a fringe lunatic. So I intentionally, held back on many areas. It was enough of a gamble to dare suggest things like non-external load leg exercises to a group of people who invariably measure their self-worth based on how much load they place on the bar in any given strength exercise.

There were those who, as expected, rejected the concepts. However, overall it was accepted far better and faster than I had expected. So in this, the second book in the *Get Buffed!*™ sequel, I am confident in going a step further.

Get Buffed! ™ II (Get More Buffed!) takes the reader to the next level. It opens up more of the information that I have yet to share with the masses. You are now ready!

The programs will be more advanced than in the original *Get Buffed!*™. I am also going to teach you how to manipulate the major variables of program design, allowing you to individualize the program for yourself. I am also going to introduce concepts and methods that I felt were not appropriate in the first book.

Get Buffed! ™ II (Get More Buffed!) takes the reader to the next level. The programs will be more advanced.

People often ask me : *"What would you write about if you wrote a sequel to the first Get Buffed!™ book?"* Believe me, it would take more than two books to exhaust myself of content! I see this second part as a complimentary sequel to the first book, as a natural progression in training and self-education regarding training.

This latest installment in the *Get Buffed!*™ range aims to take you to the next level. This book is for the readers of the original *Get Buffed!* ™ who want to **Get MORE Buffed! ™**

Enough talk – let's do it!

Introduction

Teaching you how to fish!

In the original *Get Buffed!*™ book and in this sequel to the original I provide training programs aimed to help you get bigger, stronger and leaner. However I also aim do a lot more than that. My goal is much higher, much bigger. I aim to teach you how to think. How to specifically individualize programs to better suit your needs. How to make your decisions on a daily basis about each step you take in and out of the gym throughout the day and night as it affects the training and recovery process.

I aim to teach you to balance your emotions and logic to achieve the best result possible. To trust your intuition. To have confidence that you have adequate knowledge to achieve an above average physique.

The *Get Buffed!*™ series is an extension of our educational philosophy for life – teach people how to fish, rather than simply giving them the fish.

Over time it has become more apparent to me that this is a dying concept. That many simply want the black and white answers, the fish. That there is social conditioning to believe that you don't have the power, that it is possessed only by a higher power. To question and disregard as opposed to trust your intuition.

The Get Buffed!™ series is an extension of our educational philosophy for life – teach people how to fish, rather than simply giving them the fish.

Therefore I am going to take time here to salvage your thought processes, should any of this be true in part or whole for you.

I will achieve this through addressing the following topics :

- ❑ You Don't Need More Information!
- ❑ Science Doesn't Hold the Only Key!
- ❑ You Can Trust Your Intuition!
- ❑ Action Over Procrastination – Your Choice!

You Don't Need More Information!

Why do people reach the conclusion that they need more information, or that they are waiting for science to validate it?

Have you ever thought *'I need more information before I can get started'*, or *'I wonder if science supports this?'*. Let me ask this – have you ever seen a body in a magazine from 30-50 years ago that resulted in thinking *'Gee, I wouldn't mind having a body like that!'*? I believe you may have. Did the person whose physique you admired have access to most of the information you have access to today? Of course not? Was sport science well established in those days? No! The message is very clear – you don't need that much information to get the results you are after.

I was particularly impressed to stumble upon similar sentiments expressed by a man who achieved far more than I as far as bodybuilding goes – David Draper. In his excellent book, *Brother Iron, Sister Steel* (2001, On Target Publications, CA) he wrote and I quote :

"...Get rid of the notion that you need to know more and more. The learning is in the doing. Muscle and power building are not and need never become brain surgery or astrophysics. Information beyond the ABCs and simple math only leads to confusion, doubt, controversy and frustration. These conditions distract from the wonderful world at hand and confound basic instincts and investigative courage to discover....'

So why do people go down this path? Why do people reach the conclusion that they need more information, or that they are waiting for science to validate it? I suggest a number of reasons – social conditioning that suggests that only science holds the answers, a trend towards the belief that one's own intuition is inferior, and plain old fear.

Science Doesn't Hold the Only Key!

There is a strong push within society in general and within sports science specifically that desires us all to perceive science holds the key, and in the absence of scientific validation, we cannot do anything or understand anything. How many times have your read in scientific or pseudo-scientific writings *'there is no scientific evidence to support this'*?

I say – if you were waiting for scientific validation before conducting every activity in your daily routine, you would be doing very little! Here is a different perspective to the belief that science dictates our understanding of phenomenon :

If you were waiting for scientific validation before conducting every activity in your daily routine, you would be doing very little!

"I think that in modern Western society, there seems to be a powerful cultural conditioning that is based on science. But in some instances, the basic premises and parameters set up by Western science can limit your ability to deal with certain realities. For instance, you can have the constraints of the idea that everything can be explained within the framework of a single lifetime, and you combine this with the notion that everything can and must be explained and accounted for. But when you encounter phenomenon that you cannot account for, then there's a kind of a tension created; it's almost a felling of agony."
-- Cutler, H.C., & the Dalai Lama, 1998, *The Art of Happiness*, Riverhead Books, NY,p.6.

People from all walks of life have placed 'scientific proof' in context, including philosopher Karl Popper :

"...The philosopher Karl Popper suggests that nothing can be proven correct. Scientific proof and political truth are not proof of correctness, he argues in The Open Society and Its Enemies....."
- Guppy, D., 1996, *Share Trading*, Wrightbooks, Vic.

And personal development 'guru' Anthony Robbins :

"...Now it looks as though the scientific community is finally verifying what we already found useful. There are a number of other things in this book, they'll be validating in upcoming years. But you don't have to wait for an academic researcher to confirm it for you. You can use it right away and produce the results you desire now...."
- Robbins, A., 1986, *Unlimited Power*, Ballantine Books, New York. P. 158. P. 158.

American Sales and marketing expert H. Beckwith :

The trainee (e.g. yourself, the athlete, any client of the physical preparation consultant) already possesses the answers to the training decisions.

"...Nothing said in a business meeting can match the force of any statement preceded with the words 'the research shows'. That's because research connotes something scientific. The aura of science has the remarkable ability to fool people..."
- Beckwith, H., 1997, *Selling the Invisible*, Time Warner, NY.

And industry writer Nelson Montana :

"...I love it when people cite 'studies' to me, as if they were some kind of indisputable proof. Any scientific study can only make a determination based on the science that is 'known'. At one time, doctors thought it was absurd to think that some microscopic organism can cause disease because there was no 'scientific' evidence yet available to prove it...."
- Montana, N., 1999, Feedback Letters, *Testosterone*, No. 36, Jan 22 1999.

As a final point regarding science, I believe it is worth expressing the belief that science is not always pure and objective. So don't give up the power of the decisions to something that may not be what you first thought it to be.

"For all the lip service we pay to science, everyone knows that it is commerce that runs the show. As the Spanish proverb goes, 'He who gives the bread lays down the law'. Science today typically serves the large corporate interests that fund it. In a world conceived by the financial and corporate leadership who effectively rule it, the purpose of the human being is to contribute to the economy as an increasingly efficient unit of production and as an increasingly efficient unit of consumption. The financial and corporate elite establish effective social policy, and commercially funded science gives them the technological wherewithal to execute it."
- Boldt, L.G., 1999, *The Tao of Abundance*, Penguin Books Lt., New York, p. 25.

You Can Trust Your Intuition!

Another reason that I believe drives this perception that 'more information is needed' or a delay in action is required until science delivers more conclusion is because people have been discouraged to trust their intuition.

"In a variety of ways, we've sacrificed our humanity for a sense of security in mechanical order... Having lost the confidence in intuition and instinct , we seize on the rational mind as a means of gaining control. Yet by its nature, the rational mind is always in doubt. It can never have the certainty of intuition or instinct. Isolated and defensive, mired in doubt, we turn to the machine for salvation. The culture that does not affirm the value of instinctual and intuitive intelligences must take refuge in the machine, be it the machine of dogmatic beliefs, the machine of corporate organization and the production, or the machines of consumptive pleasure."
- Boldt, L.G., 1999, The Tao of Abundance, Penguin/Arkana, NY.

When I design a training program for an athlete, the program design is more influenced by the instincts of the athlete than by rational of science. The trainee (e.g. yourself, the athlete,

Another reason that I believe drives this perception that 'more information is needed' or a delay in action is required until science delivers more conclusion is because people have been discouraged to trust their intuition.

any client of the physical preparation consultant) already possesses the answers to the training decision questions. They (and you!) just don't always know they know the answers, and don't always know how to draw them out from within. I simply help them recognize and get in touch with their instinctive responses, and reformulate it with the help of rational training knowledge. And then I give it back to them as a training program!

Action over Procrastination – Your Choice!

A final stumbling block for many is the habit of procrastination. You can find support for your procrastination in any of the above – I don't have enough information; it isn't confirmed by science; how could I trust my gut feelings? But all you are doing is finding logical reasons for your emotional limits. Procrastination involves the delay of action. Some suggest it is driven by the fear of failing, others by the feeling that one is undeserving of the possible successful outcome.

A final stumbling block for many is the habit of procrastination. You can find support for your procrastination in any of the above. But all you are doing is finding logical reasons for your emotional limits.

Either way, no action is taken. The above points are often used to legitimize this procrastination – the need for more information, or waiting for science to confirm it, and so on. A case of making an emotional decision and finding logic to validate it. One of the great delaying lines is "there is not enough scientific evidence of the effect of long-term use"....

The following is an example of this :

"Unfortunately, very little research has been conducted on the effects of long-term vitamin E supplementation and resistance training. However once that question is answered I am sure that everyone will see the benefits of taking Vitamin E."
- Craig, B.W., 2001, Vitamin E Supplementation : Does it help or hurt?, NSCA J,23(4):61-62.

The choice is yours – you can procrastinate on getting results and receive strong support from the rest of the low achieving world, or you can take action now towards achieving the physique and function you want and deserve. That's your decision. You have enough information. You don't need any more science. And yes, you hold the answers so trust you intuition!

In summary, I will never tell you what to conclude. I am simply stressing you have the power; in this book I will be giving you some tools to build your own program; and that people have been getting buffed for centuries! So there are no excuses – go out and *Get Buffed!*™

The choice is yours – you can procrastinate or you can take action now towards achieving the physique and function you want and deserve.

Chapter 1

Designing The Get Buffed!™ II Workout

Fine-tune the program to suit your needs!

In the original *Get Buffed!*™ book, published in 1999, I shared a unique four stage training program. This program included only upper and lower body workouts. There were a number of distinguishing features to this program. Firstly, the programs were unique and original. Secondly, this program (or more accurately collection of methods) had proven in the past to be very effective, and the feedback I received from those who tried it after reading this book supported the earlier findings. Thirdly, the program was a single generic program – that is, everyone did the same program. Fourthly, and finally, I chose not to over-complex the learning process, and intentionally did not include components of the workout that I in reality used at that time.

I have added more information and details about how to warm up, stretch, do control drills and abdominal training.

So what's different about the programs in this second installment of the *Get Buffed!*™ book range? Firstly, they are aimed at a higher level of trainee. Something that you can and should go onto after completing the original *Get Buffed!*™ program. Secondly, I have added more information and details about how to warm up, stretch, do control drills and abdominal training.

But most importantly, in addition to giving you generic program, I aim to teach you how to individualize that program (and any program for that matter) to better suit your individual needs. And that's powerful!

My mission is to educate you about your training decisions. This is the underlying theme of the *Get Buffed!*™ books. Not education aimed at appeasing my academic colleagues or finding the middle road of consensus – instead, my conclusions on how to train, based on my personal and professional experiences.

Before I expose you to the second generation of programs I am going to introduce you to the tools of individualization. Realistically, I am not aiming to teach you every tool of individualization. But I will introduce you to tools that are more than adequate to increase the effectiveness of your programs over and above the generic level. We are going to work with six variables, which will result in (provided my mathematics is correct!) 730 different programs and subsequent training outcomes. No, this wasn't designed as a marketing tool, but as an afterthought, wouldn't it make a great one!

For your information, the base program is a four day a week, calendar day, split routine. The program is four stages in length. That means, there are four different but connected programs. As you will learn, each stage could be a training period of somewhere between two and four weeks in length.

Throughout this program design section you are going to see reference to the terms beginner, intermediate and advanced.

So what constitutes or determines which category you fall into? There is no hard and fast rules here. However in order to give you insight into which level you could consider yourself, I have provided the following generalizations based on your 'training age'. Training age a term used to describe the number of years you have been participating in any given training activity.

Before I expose you to the second generation of programs I am going to introduce you to the tools of individualization.

Beginner   -   <1 year of continual training
Intermediate-   1-4 years of continual training
Advanced   -   >4 years of continual training

Note that these years refer to continual years of training. Once you have experienced a recent period of non-training of 6 months or more, you should at least re-commence in the earlier training level.

For example, if you had training continuously with strength training for 3 years and felt you were an intermediate level trainer, and just recently had not trained for six or more months – we would recommend you recommence with the beginner programs.

Also note that the generalized training ages (e.g. Beginner = <1 yr) are intended for those over eighteen years of age. For those younger than eighteen years of age, I advise you seek specialist advice.

The muscle done first is done best! Just like I said – simple, but don't under-estimate its power. The power is magnified over time.

These are the variables we will exploit to varying degrees :

- ❑ Body part prioritization
- ❑ Loading parameters
- ❑ Periodization models
- ❑ Rate of change
- ❑ Bilateral muscle balance
- ❑ Recovery models

Body part prioritization

There is a very simple but powerful lesson I have learned from my years of personal and practical application. The muscle done first is done best! Just like I said – simple, but don't under-estimate its power. The power is magnified over time. So if you don't see the impact over a few months, don't panic – at worst it will be obvious over a year or more! The simple example is the person who does their favorite body part first in the week and first in the workout – every time! The more this goes on for, the more the imbalance becomes!

So this is how we are going to apply a simple exploitation of this concept : I am breaking the body into three parts – upper, lower and trunk. If you are deficient in a body part, do if first in the week all the way through the final weeks. If you are balanced in these body parts, rotate them.

If you do the upper body in days 1 and 3 of the week (i.e. prioritized over lower body), then the upper body muscles will get a slightly better training effect than the lower body. Vice versa, if you do the lower body muscles on days 1 and 3, it will get a slightly better training effect than the upper body.

You can use a different sequence in each stage if you wanted to. But remember – there should be a rationale for this – don't just use variety for variety sake. Make sure the sequence reflects your needs at the time.

And as far as the most neglected 'other third' of the body goes – the abdominals or trunk - if you do them first, then they will receive priority in effort and adaptation; if done last in the workout, they will receive the lowest training effect.

The following table shows the four options I have created in relation to sequencing of the major body parts – review the options and select the one that suits your current needs the best!

Table 1 - The four options of body part prioritization and the order of sequence.

Prioritization	Body part sequence
L-U-A	Lower on A and C days, Upper on B and D days, abs last on all days
U-L-A	Upper on A and C days, Lower on B and D days, abs last on all days
A-L-U	Abs first on all days and then lower (A and C), upper (B and D)
A-U-L	Abs first on all days and then upper (A and C), lower (B and D)

Key : L=Lower body; U=Upper body; A=Abdominals or trunk

Table 2 – The four options of body part prioritization as they appear on the days of the week.

	Sun	Mon A Day	Tues B Day	Wed	Thu C Day	Fri D Day	Sat
L-U-A		Lower Abdom	Upper Abdom		Lower Abdom	Upper Abdom	
U-L-A		Upper Abdom	Lower Abdom		Upper' Abdom	Lower Abdom	
A-L-U		Abdom Lower	Abdom Upper		Abdom Lower	Abdom Upper	
A-U-L		Abdom Upper	Abdom Lower		Abdom Upper	Abdom Lower	

Now all you have to do is treat each of the four stages that make up this program as units to be manipulated, and decide how to address each stage. No, you don't have to apply the same sequence to Stage 2 and beyond because you used it in Stage 1 – you can use a different sequence in each stage if you wanted to. But remember – there should be a rationale for this – don't just use variety for variety sake. Make sure the sequence reflects your needs at the time.

You could spend years studying each of these variables. Let's just keep the process simple, allocate the bulk of this concept to training age or training goals, and pick one of the following options!

Loading parameters

One of the unique conclusions I have reached from years of participation in the training process is that the more advanced you become, the lower the repetition number that you will probably get the best response to. Put simply, 12's may have worked in the early stage, but chances are 5 or so years later, your intuition will tell you that you need to be averaging around 6 or so reps. And as time goes on, this may go down. What was once a neuro-muscular loading for you is now a hypertrophy rep, and in later years, you may find these higher reps to be totally non-response giving.

This individual response is not only a function of training age – it may also be a product of training history, training goals, sub-cultural influences, fiber type, genetics, recovery capacity and so on. You could spend years studying each of these variables – we aren't going to go there though! Let's just keep the process simple, allocate the bulk of this concept to training age or training goals, and pick one of the following options!

To cater for these powerful variables, I am going to create three options of loading parameters. You don't have to fully understand what I am doing, just what you need to do – pick one option! These are the three options I am going to create and provide throughout the four stage programs.

These thee options of loading parameters are outlined in the following table, which also shows the variables manipulated in the program design to achieve the desired effect of each option.

I am going to create three options of loading parameters. You don't have to fully understand what I am doing, just what you need to do – pick one option!

Table 3 – The three options of loading parameters and the variables manipulated to achieve the effect.

Option	Variables Manipulated to Achieve Effect		
	Sequence	Reps (and therefore loading)	Rest periods
Hypertrophy dominant goals; and/or early training age	Pre-fatigue in hypertrophy phases	Higher numbers and or longer time under tension	Shorter, and in hypertrophy phases, more use of tri and super sets
Balance between hypertrophy-neural goals; and/or intermediate training age	A mix of pre-fatigue and conventional sequence in hypertrophy phases	Medium numbers and / or medium time under tension	Medium
Neural dominant goals; and/or advanced training age	Conventional in hypertrophy phases	Lower numbers and or shorter time under tension	Longer, including in hypertrophy phases

If you are still unsure, you can easily decide which combination is most suited to you now based on your recent training experiences.

Periodization models

The subject of periodization has gone from a coach's tool to a writer's tool along with the subsequent confusion. Put simply, periodization simply means to plan. There is really no such thing as the Russian way, or the American way. There may be patterns of commonality within regions or countries, but the concept of periodization doesn't start and stop in Russia. Certain Russian sport scientist certainly made a massive contribution and for this they should be acknowledged. But to assume that the concept of planning is exclusive to Russia and Russian methods – that's simply a marketing scam. I call it Soviet scam! Anyone who wanted to market themselves claims they had traveled to Russia and returned with the 'secrets'!

There is really no such thing as the Russian way, or the American way. There may be patterns of commonality within regions or countries, but the concept of planning doesn't start and stop in Russia.

Now we have demystified the concept, lets work it! Again in the interests of simplicity, I present two options. I call them linear and alternating. No, they are not the only ones, but don't throw the baby out with the bathwater – if they work for you, use them, trendy or not!

Linear periodization involves a progressive reduction in one variable (e.g. reps) and an inverse change in another variable (e.g. load). Most commonly, a program will start with high reps, low load, and then trend in the other direction. The benefit of linear periodization is that you can work towards your optimal loading in a progressive manner. The downside is that at the start you may be de-training the effects you get at the end, and at the end you may be de-training the effects you may get at the start. Put the downsides on the shelf for the moment – if you are what I would call a beginner or intermediate trainer, this will work. And it may even work at times in an advanced trainer. (see example below)

*Table 4 - An example of **linear periodization**.*

Reps

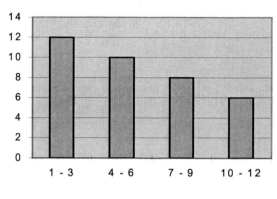

Week No.s

Alternating periodization involves taking a more significant jump up and down the reps and loading. The benefits of alternating periodization is that you get more frequent exposure to the varying stimulus, and thus less likely to detrain any of them. The downside is that you need to be experienced in load selection, or you may not work near optimal loading – the loading jumps around a lot more. As a beginner I wouldn't rush into using alternating periodization, but as an advanced trainer it is more likely to work for you. Intermediate trainers can go either way. (see example below)

*Table 5 - An example of **alternating periodization**.*

Reps

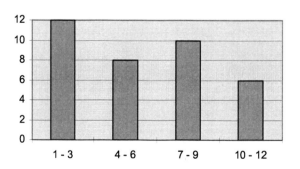

In this four stage program I will present them in either of the above – all you need to do is pick up on that and change it around. For example, if I say that a program is going to be a linear program like this :

Table 6 – Sample average reps in a linear periodized program.

Sample Average Reps			
Stage 1	Stage 2	Stage 3	Stage 4
10-20	8-15	6-10	4-8

And you want to make it into an alternating program, do the four stages in this order :

As a beginner I wouldn't rush into using alternating periodization, but as an advanced trainer it is more likely to work for you.

Table 7 – How to change a generic linear periodization program into an alternated periodization program.

Sample Average Reps			
Stage 1	Stage 3	Stage 2	Stage 4
10-20	6-10	8-15	4-8

Conversely, if I present the four stage program as an alternating program, such as this :

Table 8 – Sample average reps in an alternating periodized program.

Sample Average Reps			
Stage 1	Stage 2	Stage 3	Stage 4
10-20	6-10	8-15	4-8

And if you want to make it into a linear program, do the four stages in this order :

Table 9 – How to change a generic alternating periodization program into a linear periodization program.

Sample Average Reps			
Stage 1	Stage 3	Stage 2	Stage 4
10-20	8-15	6-10	4-8

Don't be sucked into using an alternating or more exotic form or periodization just because it is exotic – the only thing that should matter to you is the result.

Don't be sucked into using an alternating or more exotic form or periodization just because it is exotic – the only thing that should matter to you is the result, and you need to apply your intuition and rationale, not your emotions in making this decision.

Rate of change

How many weeks you should stay on the one program can be influenced by a lot of variables, but I am going to focus on the 20% that give 80% of the impact. These include rate of adaptation and exposure to loading.

An experienced person, a person closer to their possible ceiling of possibilities, has less room for improvement, and therefore can plateau out more quickly. A relative novice, on the other hand, who has lots of room between their current capacities and their ceiling of possibilities, may experience greater improvement and this improvement may continue over a longer period of time. Literally interpreted, the less experienced you are relative to any given exercise or muscle group, the longer you can and should stay on a program. Conversely, the more experienced you are, the shorter your exposure should be. When I say program, I am in particular referring to sets, reps, rest period, speed of movement and exercises. These are the major variables that when manipulated, constitute a 'new program'.

The other major influencing variable on rate of change is exposure to intensity. If you are exposed to loading closer to your current maximum early in a program, the time frame you will probably benefit from staying on that program is diminished. This may be because you are taken closer to your ceiling earlier, or because it creates earlier onset of residual fatigue – or more likely, both. As I say, we just need to work out what to do – we can leave the why's to those who dedicate their life to seeking these answers.

So how do you know which rate of change to use? Most importantly, learn from your experiences. If you have seen a pattern of improvement for 'x' number of weeks followed by a sudden reduction or halting of improvement, take note of this pattern. The critical variable is intensity. If you change the intensity from what you did in those examples that gave you insight, you move the goal posts. So I say this – all things being equal (i.e. if you use the same intensity exposure and progression you did previously), you can expect to plateau in 'x' weeks.

If you are exposed to loading closer to your current maximum early in a program, the time frame you will probably benefit from staying on that program is diminished.

The most common successful numbers of weeks I have seen and used for adult clients (I say adult as kids can often use longer periods) is 4, 3 and 2 – going from least experienced to most experienced. So if I say this program is a three (3) weeks per stage program, and your intuition tells you to use 2 or 4 weeks – do so!

I would encourage you however to apply my progressive intensity models as follows :

Table 10 – Progressive application of intensity for the less experienced lifter, or those wishing to develop the load capacity slowly.

Week No	Key Words	Example %age loading
1	Focus on technique Easy loading No high level fatigue No failure	80-85% of previous RM
2	Maintain technical focus Medium loading No failure	85-90% of previous RM
3	Maintain technique as load rises Higher level of fatigue No failure	95-100% or previous RM
4	Focus on loading with minimal diminishment of technique Highest level of fatigue short of failing Don't aim to fail but may occur	100-105% or previous RM

So how do you know which rate of change to use? Most importantly, learn from your experiences.

Table 11 – Progressive application of intensity for intermediate lifter.

Week No	Key Words	Example %age loading
1	Focus on technique Medium loading No failure	85-90% of previous RM
2	Maintain technique as load rises Higher level of fatigue No failure	95-100% or previous RM
3	Focus on loading with minimal diminishment of technique Highest level of fatigue short of failing Don't aim to fail but may occur	100-105% or previous RM

Remember, I am not telling you what to do – just giving you some guidance – you decide, and you analysis objectively at the end as to the effectiveness of your decision.

Table 12 – Progressive application of intensity for advanced lifter.

Week No	Key Words	Example %age loading
1	Focus on technique Higher level of fatigue No failure	95-100% or previous RM
2	Focus on loading with minimal diminishment of technique Highest level of fatigue short of failing Don't aim to fail but may occur	100-105% or previous RM

These rates of change guidelines are just that guidelines – I know elite lifters who don't change much over 12 weeks! Remember, I am not telling you what to do – just giving you some guidance – you decide, and you analysis objectively at the end as to the effectiveness of your decision.

Bilateral muscle balance

Bilateral muscle balance in this case refers to equal strength between right and left sides or limbs. Very few people are truly balanced in this area. So this is a very strong case of the needs of individuals being met. If you use a barbell, those bilateral imbalances are not only ignored, they may become worse – because your strong side can do more of the work and you sometimes don't even realize it.

You may have such a significant imbalance say between your right and left arms, that you should NEVER (or at least not until the imbalance is corrected) use a barbell.

You may have such a significant imbalance say between your right and left arms, that you should NEVER (or at least not until the imbalance is corrected) use a barbell. Yet you may see a program that says 'barbell whatever', and literally interpret it – against your best interests. I want to encourage you to do this – even where I have not provided a unilateral movement, if you know it is not in your best interests to be using a barbell or similar bilateral device- don't! Find a suitable unilateral option!

Recovery models

This concept of recovery or half-recovery weeks is nothing new – at least in training literature. It is a sound training principle applied with regular monotony in most high level sports training programs. Why it has not been so applied in general strength training is not as clear. Is it the lack of education? Or is lack of control of emotions? (how could I take a week off...my biceps would fall off!). Maybe it is the opportunity to simply raise the chemical intake when fatigue sets in! Whatever, most people when reminiscing about their training past will express key words that tell me instinctively where they should place their recovery weeks. Statements like : "*I go really well for 3 weeks then I crash*" – take a recovery week after every 3 weeks of training!

Sounds simple? It is! Either take the recovery week or modify your exposure to loading along the progressive exposure to intensity model I promote – or both. Either way, you won't know until you have tried it – and as many smart coaches now know (and I think we can credit Charlie Francis amongst others for this) *'if in doubt do less'*!

I have created five (5) options that suit a variety of rate of change combinations, and these are outlined below. To help determine whether the rest week should be a full or half recovery week, read the relevant section in the original *Get Buffed! ™* book.

Either take the recovery week or modify your exposure to loading along the progressive exposure to intensity model I promote – or both.

Table 13 – Options in recovery weeks.

Option	Total weeks in program if using 4 stages	Rate of change combinations it suits
3+1	16 wks	3 week stages
4+1	20 wks	4 week or 2 x 2 week stages
6+1	14 wks	2 x 3 week stages
8+1	9 wks	4 x 2 week stages
12+1	13 wks	4 x 2 wk blocks straight

Which one do you use? Pick one of them and learn from doing! The one thing I can say for sure – if you don't use one of the above or something very similar you may be short-changing yourself.

Conclusion

By now you should have made a decision as to which option you are going to use within the six variables of individualization that have been identified.

Pick one of them and learn from doing!

Table 14 – A summary of all the individual variables and their options for you to manipulate.

Individualization Variables	Options				
	1	2	3	4	5
Body part	L-U-A	U-L-A	A-L-U	A-U-L	
Loading parameters	Hyper-trophy/ Lower training age	Hyper-trophy-neural /Medium training age	Neural / Ad-vanced training age		
Periodization model	Linear	Alternat-ing			
Rate of change	4 weeks	3 weeks	2 weeks		
Bilateral muscle balance	Unilateral	Bilateral			
Recovery models	3+1	4+1	6+1	8+1	12+1

Chapter 2
Additional Training

What impact will it have?

The prior chapter was totally focused on strength training. You may at any time want to or need to do additional training. The starting point in this discussion is that any training of a different nature will dilute the specific adaptation of the *Get Buffed!*™ program. But this is not necessarily good or bad. That depends on your goals. I just want to make it clear – if you allocate your effort and recovery to training of a mixed adaptations, you will get a mixed result. All you need to decide is if the total result of training is consistent with your overall short and long term goals.

Any training of a different nature will dilute the specific adaptation of the Get Buffed!™ program.

Here are some common situations that result in people wanting to or needing to do additional, non-strength training:

- Lowering Body Fat
- Sporting Needs
- Other Physical Pursuit
- Other Recreational Pursuits

Lowering Body Fat

Before deciding to use training to lower body fat, consider the two major elements – training and nutrition. Where the additional training provides you with a specific benefit other than energy expenditure, using training as the dominant contributor is fine. When the additional training has little or negative benefit, you should be putting in a bigger effort to get the result through diet.

Experts and pseudo-experts love to debate the exercise vs. diet combination, and further which type of exercise is most effective – high intensity or low intensity. As American philosopher Jim Rohn says, *"You can study the roots or pick the fruit"*. By now you may have realized that I am from the school of 'pick the fruit'!

Bottom line is that body fat is more of an issue in a society that has been mechanized and automated. If we were walking or riding bikes more etc., we probably wouldn't be having this discussion. I have worked with so many athletes whose body fat was low from their specific sports training despite an 'eat what you want' approach to nutrition. Exercise is a powerful contributor to lower body fat!

When the additional training has little or negative benefit, you should be putting in a bigger effort to get the result through diet.

If you are going to use additional training to lower body fat, and there are specific benefits consistent with your goals from doing this activity, you probably know what to do. If you are going to use what I call non-specific exercise to contribute to lowering your body fat – activity that you have no need or benefit from the specific training adaptation, check out these guidelines.

- Use low intensity training. Remember this is not about what burns the most calories. This is about non-specific additional training and my goal is to minimize the downside of that training. I believe that low intensity training interferes less with the recovery and adaptation to the training effect of strength training.
- Longer duration or higher frequency is even better. When you are wanting to accelerate the effect on body fat of non-specific non-weight training, look to do it longer or more often. You can do both without

interfering with the recovery process extensively – provided it is low intensity?

- What is low intensity? Some would suggest a heart rate and if you are heart rate included I would say no higher than about 120 b/m. The challenge with that is some could get up from a chair and achieve that whilst other would need to sprint 100 meters to get it up there! So a more accurate yet subjective guideline would be to say a comfortable, just sweating, level of work. Where you can still hold conversation but are sweating.
- What type of exercise? Walking and cycling are my pick. Running is an option but more interfering with the recovery process, and swimming is far too demanding on the upper body recovery and adaptation to strength training. Unless you were using say kickboard and flippers or a similar combination.
- What time of day? I suspect earlier in the day the better, however the relative benefits of this may not be worth you changing your day up for.

You will notice that in this *Get Buffed!™* program I have allowed for two days a week of additional training (Wednesday and Saturday) that also double up as a warm up for an extended stretching session. Additionally, you have your pre-training warm up activity, the duration of which can be manipulated by yourself should you want to extend it to burn more energy.

Once your knowledge of training exceeds your coaches, which is not difficult in most cases, feel free to make informed decisions. Stand your ground. Remember it is your body, your career.

Sporting Needs

Many will be involved in sports that require additional non-strength training. I will assume you have no choice but to participate. However from my experience and observations, most training recommendations of coaches and strength & conditioning coaches include ineffective and excessive volume training. Once your knowledge of training exceeds your coaches, which is not difficult in most cases, feel free to make informed decisions. Stand your ground. Remember it is your body, your career. You are responsible for the outcome so don't give away the power!

In relation to the non-strength training component that you deem necessary and must be done, I make the following suggestions :

- Ask yourself again – is the training really necessary? Is it really beneficial? What would be the impact of not doing it or doing less of it? You may be surprised by the answer! If in doubt, experiment, but do so with an objective mind.
- Work your strength training around the other training. When you cannot modify the training type, content and timing, make sure you modify your strength training program to take that into account. Over-training achieves nothing. If in doubt, do less. You certainly should not be doing a four-day a week strength training program if you are in a sports program that involves multiple week training in the specific sporting activity or other non-strength training sessions.
- Look to have a fantastic GPP! The GPP is the General Preparatory Phase. This is the athlete's annual opportunity to *Get Buffed!*™. Don't blow it. Look to get as much control of this phase as possible. If you are in an energy based sport and train all year round, minimize your energy system training in this phase and prioritize your strength training!

If you are in an energy based sport and train all year round, minimize your energy system training in the GPP and prioritize your strength training!

Other Physical Pursuit

Many of you will be involved in other intense but not necessarily competitive activities, such as martial arts training. This, as in sports training (above) or recreation training (below), provide specific adaptations that are consistent with your goals – but don't necessarily support the specific goal of getting bigger, stronger and leaner. It's simply a trade-off, one that I support – I am not into looking good as the sole goal. I prefer a body that can perform, not just appear to be able to perform!

My suggestions for those of you pursing non-competitive intense non-strength training are similar to those in competitive sports training. Here are a few more :

- Most martial artist over train their specific sport. This provides neither a superior martial arts adaptation nor strength training adaptation. Find out what is really needed to achieve your goals in your specific training and don't overstep that. Generally speaking most fighters could halve their training and they would still be over training!
- Create our own GPP. In sports, most athletes are forced into a GPP, except those on a year-round competitive calendar. In individual non-competitive sports, you need to enforce on yourself. Have 2-4 months where strength training dominates, and you do very little of the other training e.g. martial arts training.

You quite simply need to decide how much adaptation you wish to get from strength training and how much from your recreational activity.

Other Recreational Pursuits

Surprisingly, despite the lack of structure and regularity in training sessions of these types, recreational pursuits can negate *Get Buffed!*™ training. Take surfing for example – the upper body muscular and total body neural and metabolic fatigue can be devastating! In fact, any upper body dominant activity such as kayaking and rock climbing, if performed excessively, will negate adaptations to strength training.

You quite simply need to decide how much adaptation you wish to get from strength training and how much from your recreational activity. Again, the above guidelines for sports training apply, and I add :

- Create your own GPP. It may be best to have a 2-4 month period of the year once or two 1-2 month periods of the year where you do minimal if any of your recreational activity and prioritize strength training.
- So when you are prioritizing your recreational activity, be prepared to maintain what *Get Buffed!*™ adaptations you have through lower volume strength training.

It may be best to have a 2-4 month period of the year once or two 1-2 month periods of the year where you do minimal if any of your recreational activity and prioritize strength training.

Chapter 3
The Recovery Process

The other half of the training equation!

I have taught throughout the *Get Buffed!*™ series that you will only see the training effect after you recover from the training. That the training effect is a combination of training and recovery, and therefore your focus and attention to the recovery process is as important as your focus and attention on the training process.

The training effect is a combination of training and recovery, and therefore your focus and attention to the recovery process is as important as your focus and attention on the training process.

Training takes or depletes. It disrupts homeostasis, destroys tissues. The degree of damage you inflict needs to be in context of your recovery ability. Exceed it at your peril. The replacement or replenishment, known as the recovery process, is not rigid. You can alter it, although age and stress is amongst the more powerful forces that will work against you. You can alter it through various means including nutrition, supplements, drugs, sleep/rest etc. If you want to train harder, longer or more often, be prepared to spend time and energy learning about and implementing ways to enhance recovery. This focus on recovery enhancement is often the difference between winning and losing.

I have also taught that lack of response to training is more often the cause of over-training than any other factor. Over-training occurs when one is exposed to a subsequent bout of training before recovering from the previous one. When this occurs a number of times in a row, you start to see more obvious signs of over-training. Mainstream literature and science has traditionally focused on these symptoms rather than the prevention of them. You often read the words 'over-training syndrome' and 'planned over-training'. There is no need for this – if you are in control of the training and recovery process, if you train to preset levels, and recover in pre-planned ways, you don't need to know anything about over-training 'syndromes'!

Now there are two parts to this – training and recover. So in reality, you can over train, or you can under recover. Bottom line is, you need to know how far you should push the training, based on your anticipated recovery ability – taking into account the recovery capacity you possess and the methods you will implement.

In this chapter I will be addressing :

- ❑ Training Decisions Based on Frequency and Recovery
- ❑ Monitoring Over-training
- ❑ Recovery Methods

You need to know how far you should push the training, based on your anticipated recovery ability – taking into account the recovery capacity you possess and the methods you will implement.

Training Decisions Based on Frequency and Recovery

Now in relation to training frequency, you can pre-determine days and stick to them, as I have done in the *Get Buffed!*™ training series, or you can train when you are recovered, whenever that is. They both work, and they both have downsides. Why have I gone with a fixed training day? I have done this because I want to apply discipline and pattern to your life. Humans are creatures of habit, and when you have a habit it is best to stick to it. Additionally, as we live in a society that respects a calendar week, it is best for the average person to work to a calendar cycle.

Now I am not saying this is the only way to write programs, or necessarily the best. I do believe that for the majority of you it will be the best. Your challenge is to make decisions in a training session about how much to do, how hard to go – with the knowledge of your recovery capacity and recovery methods you will implement – so that by the time you return to the gym next, you will be recovered. So that the next time you repeat this workout, usually in a week's time, you will be able to do it better.

If for whatever reason you get into the next workout and you realize that you have not recovered, you have two choices – walk out or reduce the volume and the degree of increment in the load. Provided you can see some increment in at least one work set, I want you to do this and then cut the volume short. So that the next time you come back to do the same workout you can do more – you have obviously improved.

Now you can walk out without training if you need to. If you made serious errors in judgment in the prior workout, or if life took an unexpected twist (e.g. you didn't get much sleep the night before) – and if you cannot see an increment in load ability or if you felt you were risking injury – then I want you to go home!

If you get into the next workout and you realize that you have not recovered, you have two choices – walk out or reduce the volume and the degree of increment in the load.

You have this flexibility. You make the decisions. Your goal should be to get better from week to week but if you are not seeing that, cut back! Don't ignore it or pretend it isn't happening. The beauty of strength training is that it is so measurable!

Monitoring Recovery

So how do I recommend you monitor recovery? Generally speaking I don't like to use only one indicator to monitor recovery. In the most advanced situations, such as recovering a professional athlete who has presented him/her self to me with chronic fatigue, I monitor up to ten variables, including :

- Sleep
- Bodyweight
- Resting heart-rate
- Energy levels
- Desire to train
- Appetite
- Skill level
- Flexibility/stiffness
- Facial freshness
- Work Capacity

The general assessment of recovery I use involves asking the following questions :

If your recovery status is such that it is affecting your sleep, then the sleep disturbance from this over-training condition will further damage your recovery status.

✓ Did you feel stronger in every week?
✓ Did you remain keen to train in every week?
✓ If your goal was to put on weight did it happen?
✓ Are you sleeping well?
✓ How are your moods?

If I had to nominate the single best indicator, I would suggest sleep. This is how I monitor sleep as an indicator of recovery. I ask the following three questions :

1. Did you go to sleep easily?
2. Did you sleep well?
3. How did you feel when you woke up?

The amazing thing about sleep is the way it acts in a vicious cycle. If your recovery status is such that it is affecting your sleep (e.g. you are over-training), then the sleep disturbance from this over-training condition will further damage your recovery status. The key to minimizing this damage is to recognize it as early as possible, and take effective steps to knock it on the head. These steps will include reduction of training, as well as improving current recovery methods, and introducing new recovery methods. I regularly face the task of counseling athletes with sleep disorders because this early intervention was not implemented. No matter when it occurs, intervention is necessary to return the athlete to an optimal sleep pattern.

Recovery Methods

There are many methods you can implement as part of your recovery methods. I will focus on the following ones. I have chosen them because I believe they are cost-effective and easy to implement. There is no excuse or reason why all of you cannot be implementing them!

- o Nutrition
- o Sleep Management
- o Connective Tissue Status
- o Lifestyle

Nutrition

Nutrition is responsible for replacing energy in the body, and controlling hormone release.

In relation to the nutritional role of replacing energy to enhance recovery, some of my recommendations include :

- Eat breakfast! This is a meal that 'breaks the fast'. Extending that fast can be very catabolic (i.e. causes more muscle tissue damage).
- Never experience hunger pains. This is a message from the body that you have starved it of nutrition, and that it has begun to 'rob from Peter to give to Paul'. It has commenced activities such as amino acid stealing – taking from certain areas such as muscle and giving to more vital organs. This is catabolic!
- Don't train hungry, unless your goal is to lose weight and possibly size! You enter the workout in a potentially catabolic state and therefore the degree of post-training catabolism (which is normal) will be

Don't train hungry, unless your goal is to lose weight and possibly size!

greater than normal. Your last meal should be such that you would not need your next meal until some time after training.

- Even if you were not hungry before training, you need to anticipate if you would get hungry during training. If so, eat something before or during training you can tolerate, or put back training so you can eat!
- Never miss your post-training intake! The sooner you get this in after training the better. I like it to happen within 15 minutes of the end of the workout. Whether it is protein or carb dominant depends on the contents of your prior intake and your goals.
- Follow up your post-training intake with a meal, within the hour!
- Consider supplements such as antioxidants and minerals and creatine amongst others. Antioxidants protect the cells from the damage caused by free radicals. Creatine accelerates cellular hydration and energy replacement.
- If you find any foods or supplements support your immune system, you should also consider them e.g. colostrum, garlic, selected anti-oxidants, etc.

Never miss your post-training intake! The sooner you get this in after training the better. I like it to happen within 15 minutes of the end of the workout.

In relation to the role of nutrition in controlling hormone release for recovery, some of my recommendations include :

- Elevate glycogen levels immediately post training, to inhibit the release of the cortisol hormone, known for its role in catabolism (breaking down of muscle).
- Ensure appropriate nutrition in the hours after training to ensure the cortisol release does not become too extensive.

There is the possible consideration of using selective amino acids to enhance natural growth hormone release, but I hesitate to go down that path with you at this level because of the uncertainty that they are able to elevate your GH significantly enough to make a difference.

Sleep Management

Sleep is incredibly important in the training process with its contribution to recovery. I believe that it is an area of training that is still underdone. I like the concept of the training triangle – eating, sleeping and training! Here are some tips for getting a good night's sleep :

- Get as many hours before midnight as you can. There is a belief that an hour before midnight is worth two hours of after mid-night sleep.
- Get in a pattern of sleep – when you go to bed and when you get up. When you change this pattern, irrespective of if you actually get more sleep, it can negatively impact on recovery.
- Make your room dark and noise free – that means using dark curtains and closing windows and doors (but of course maintain appropriate room temperature!) Your sleep hormone release may be better in a darker environment.
- Engage in a relaxing activity before turning the lights out – there is nothing worse than going to bed fired up, overly excited or similar. Some find a warm bath effective, and some may find reading a book for 10-20 minutes may help them feel drowsy. It needs to be an appropriate book – not that that is too compelling! If you turn the lights out when the eyes say no more reading, you will be better positioned to fall asleep quickly!
- Once the lights are out stay on your back until you find you are about to go to sleep and then roll to one side.
- I do support the use of sleep inducers when you are struggling to go to sleep. I have found the following effective : melatonin in particular, or some other form of magnesium. I recommend you use a magnesium

Get as many hours before midnight as you can. There is a belief that an hour before midnight is worth two hours of after mid-night sleep.

supplement most nights. In special sleep challenged situations, I recommend the use of melatonin. Situations you may find this useful include when training related fatigue is disturbing your sleep; or if you work late and have only limited hours sleep; or if you are in a new time zone and struggling to get to sleep. If you are going through a period of struggling to go to sleep I would recommend them but generally speaking I would not use melatonin or other prescription sleep inducers for more than 3 nights in a row. I don't like becoming reliant on them.

- As indicated above, I recommend you use nightly a high dose multi-mineral that includes magnesium. The chelated minerals in Usana's 'Essentials' (multi vitamin/mineral) pack is excellent for this. The better quality sleep that these kind of supplements create go a long way to enhancing recovery from training. Remember, if most of your growth hormone release and muscle recovery occurs during sleep, you want the best sleep quality possible! Over and above the anti-oxidant protection of the cells, these sleep enhancement from a high-dose high-quality multi-vitamin/mineral is critical. For more information on the vitamins, check out www.unitoday.net/king.

- If you use an alarm clock to wake up in the morning, your first few hours of the day may not be as good as they could be when compared to a situation where you woke naturally. The body can wake naturally, in particular in response to light. However due to lifestyles (e.g. work etc.) many need or lead a life where they need to use an alarm. I prefer not to. You can wake up when you need to without one, and naturally. This works provided you don't get too run down, in which case your body can sleep through. Also, if I had a critical appointment or a job where punctuality was of the highest priority, I understand the need for an alarm.

- The ideal situation is to go to bed early and rise early. The pattern of the sun going down at the end of the day and rising the next day is a message – you should

If you use an alarm clock to wake up your first few hours of the day may not good as they could when compared to a situation where you woke naturally.

work with it, not against it. As eccentric as it sounds, this is the ideal lifestyle for getting buffed!

Connective Tissue Status

Connective tissue, including muscle tissue, changes as a result of the training. The temperature and tension is raised, and the tissue shortened. This state is less conducive to optimal muscle function, and inhibits fluid flow and nerve transmission. If you don't return the connective tissue to it's optimal condition, your adaptation is inhibited. The longer you take to return it, the slower the recovery process. So your goal, if you wish to optimize the recovery contribution of this method, is to return the tissue to optimal condition as soon as possible.

Connective tissue, including muscle tissue, changes as a result of the training. The temperature and tension is raised, and the tissue shortened. This state is less conducive to optimal muscle function, and inhibits fluid flow and nerve transmission.

The main techniques I recommend at this level include :

- **Temperature reduction** : The aim of this activity is to lower the body temperature. The theory here is that an elevated temperature has catabolic potential, and you want to bring this down as soon as possible. This can be as simple as getting in the shower. Or if you are training in a hot environment, resting in a cooler environment. One of my favorites is relaxing in a swimming pool.

- **Neural firing alteration** : The aim of this activity is to reduce the nervous system to a lower setting. The theory here is that as a result of training it's firing level is elevated, causing a drain of nerve chemicals, and holding connective tissue at higher tension levels due to above normal neural tension.

  There are many ways to address this, and in fact all the methods discussed in this section contribute. Specifically, exposing oneself to a relaxing environment and activity is the best, cheapest and simplest. Again, lying around the pool is fantastic. Alternatively, chilling out in the locker room or in the gym café or a local café. Another great alternative that has deep support in Eastern European training literature is exposure to salt water and sea breeze, or mountain fresh air – exposure to calming elements of nature. There is added benefits, including the absorption of vitamins from the sun etc. These have long been recognized in strength training literature.

- **Temperature contrasting** : This technique has potential to lower temperature and neural firing, with the added bonus of flushing the fluid systems of the body. The theory is that this will accelerate the removal of waste products. This may be as simple as alternating between hot and cold in a shower. In a more advanced environment, alternating between a cold or plunge pool and a warmer pool or spa.

This may be as simple as alternating between hot and cold in a shower. In a more advanced environment, alternating between a cold or plunge pool and a warmer pool or spa.

- **Stretching** : Stretching is the major contributor to returning connective tissue to optimum. This is an extremely powerful recovery method, although not given the extent of credit in literature that it deserves. And definitely not given this priority in practical application across the world. But I suggest that this will change. Don't wait for everyone else to work it out. In this *Get Buffed!*™ program, I have allocated a Wednesday and Saturday training session to this activity. Ensure it is focused and relaxed. A great chance to apply a meditative approach. In addition to lengthening connective tissue, you can lower neural tension and muscular tension.

- **Massage** : Massage is not as cost-effective as your stretching, but does provide a unique benefit. Massage can lower tension in connective tissue very effectively, and specifically in areas that are less responsive to stretching. For example, the ITB (tissue on the outside of the upper thigh) responds more to tension reduction through massage than stretching, generally speaking.

Lifestyle

Recovery is not complete without consideration of lifestyle. For the best results in training, your lifestyle needs to be optimal. Here are some lifestyle issues that you need to consider :

- **Minimize stress** : stress, irrespective of its source, is catabolic. This is counterproductive to getting the best possible training effect from your *Get Buffed!*™ program. If you are not prepared to live a lifestyle where you metabolism can slow down, don't expect above average hypertrophy!
- **Minimize or eliminate drugs** : they interfere with the body's homeostasis. Some more so than others. This includes alcohol!
- **Get regular sleep** : don't expect to be a night party animal and optimize the training effect.

I have a saying that you can do what you want until you are 21 – and after that, if you haven't got smart about your training – you will be in trouble!

If you are young and don't have a lifestyle that reflects the above and yet seem to get away with it, don't get comfortable. Once you hit an age somewhere between your early to mid twenties, you will probably not get away with this sub-optimal lifestyle. In fact, I have a saying that you can do what you want until you are 21 – and after that, if you haven't got smart about your training – you will be in trouble! Initially (say from 22-25 years of age) you will notice a plateau. After that you will notice a reduction in capacity and recovery. So get organized!

Chapter 4

Eating to Get Buffed!™

Fueling the furnace!

One area that I feel the 'iron game' has led in the total training process is in the area of nutrition. Strength trainees have historically been more committed to exploring this aspect of the training triangle (eat, sleep, train) than most other sports persons. Consequently, there is no shortage of literature on this topic. The flipside of this is that because the nutritional industry has always had strong commercial interests, you need to always review the concepts from a more objective manner than the marketing would have you.

My belief is that it takes about three years in the market for the true effect of a new concept or supplement to be assessed.

There are other aspects of nutrition I want to counsel you on. Being on the cutting edge of nutritional science, as is the strength training industry in general, has its upsides and downsides. The upsides is you get to hear about latest developments first. The downside is you are the guinea pig! My belief is that it takes about three years in the market for the true effect of a new concept or supplement to be assessed. In this time you have a large sample size of subjects (people like you willing to trial the latest offering), and you need this time or similar for the marketing and placebo affect to wear off!

Therefore you need to realize that you may want to be cautious at coming to a conclusion about the cause-effect relationship of new nutritional concepts and products. You need to allow time to dilute the inescapable impact of marketing alone.

If you are one of those who jumps into new concepts and products as soon as they become available, the fact you are a guinea pig is not bad. It's actually good – you are making a contribution to the body of knowledge! Just understand that you are engaging in the risk that you may have been wasting your time and money. As long as you understand that, everyone will be happy!

The final word of caution is there is a strong commercial need in the nutrition industry to recreate an old concept or product with a different twist each year, especially if there is not a new concept or product to promote. To ensure continued high sales, there is pressure to give you something new – even if only by changing the label!

Creatine is one of the few product breakthroughs I have witnessed, but did taking it with the grape juice make that much of a difference?

In my training career, I have seen relatively little true breakthroughs or innovations in concepts and products. In other words most of what I have seen has been hyped up trash. The understanding and appreciation of fats was one of the few conceptual breakthroughs. Creatine is one of the few product breakthroughs I have witnessed, but did taking it with the grape juice make that much of a difference? Glucosamine is another – but does taking it with chondroitin make it better? Maybe, maybe not.

What I want to do now is to give you some solid principles of eating to *Get Buffed!™* that I have formed over the years. I will leave the more complex theories to those more appropriately qualified to share them. I do enjoy their information. I simply want to give you some foundational guidelines to which you can add any manner of concepts and products from the ever-growing menu of nutritional and nutritional supplement information!

In this chapter I will address :

- ❏ Going Beyond the RDA's
- ❏ Eating to Recover
- ❏ Eating to Manipulate Hormones
- ❏ Nutrition Options – Volume and Type
- ❏ Eating to Get Bigger
- ❏ Eating to Get Stronger
- ❏ Eating to Get Leaner
- ❏ The Forgotten Nutrients

Going Beyond the RDA's

Hopefully some of you will be so young you won't remember the RDAs! That is, the 'Recommended Dietary Allowances', the US government supported 'rubber stamp' of what you need to eat. Few know that the aim of the RDA's was to prevent scurvy or rickets (do you know anyone who has suffered from this?) and similar nutritional deficiency conditions. Or that these guidelines were introduced in the 1940s! Or that these guidelines were based on the <u>minimum criteria necessary to prevent acute nutritional deficiencies!</u>

Few know that the aim of the RDA's was to prevent scurvy or rickets; or that these guidelines were introduced in the 1940s!

Anyway, I assume you want to know what you need to do for optimal performance and health, not minimal health!

Just in case any of you have been around long enough to possess any carryover influence from that restricted era, I have provided insights into how the attitude towards protein was negatively affected by the attachment by mainstream to these RDAs.

Many of you would be aware that prior to about 1990 it was extremely rare to see any mainstream nutritionist or scientist recommend anything above the USA Recommended Dietary Allowance (RDA) of 0.7 gms of protein per kilogram of bodyweight.

The mainstream consensus of the 1980's is reflected in nutritional text (e.g. (Williams, M.H., 1983, *Nutrition for Sport and Fitness*, WCB, Iowa, USA) that taught that those over 19 years of age required 0.8 gms of protein per kg of bodyweight. The author went on further to say that *"the minimum necessary intake of protein is much less than the RDA..."*, that the RDA's were actually adjusted upwards to take into account the variability in the biological quality of protein!

This author did recognize the existence of theories supporting higher intake of protein but aimed to debunk them.

Fortunately there were scientists even during the 1980s that were reaching and teaching a different opinion to this mainstream conservative approach, but it would not be likely that the average man on the street would be exposed to this 'radical' approach in that decade.

"...we suggest that athletes consume 1.8-2.0g of protein/kilogram of bodyweight/day...."
- Lemon, P.W, Yarasheski, K.E., and Dolny, D.G., 1984, The importance of protein for athletes, *Sports Medicine*, 1:474-484.

So what were the American strength and conditioning fraternity being taught in the late 1980s?

"...RDAs for protein are calculated at two standard deviations beyond the average requirement. This extrapolation then includes virtually all the population regardless of variance in physical activity behaviors...to date there is insufficient evidence to suggest that the well-conditioned strength or endurance athlete needs to alter what is now considered a healthy diet for the American population.."

It gets better :

"...In the strength and conditioning community, the conventional wisdom that athletes need additional protein beyond that provided

> *Fortunately there were scientists even during the 1980s that were reaching and teaching a different opinion to this mainstream conservative approach.*

by normal dietary practices is due in part to simply myth, to poorly designed studies given undue credit ...."
- Sargent, R.G., 1988, Protein needs for the athlete, *NSCA J, 10(4):53-55.*

The above author did recognize support for higher protein intake but appeared to place a foot either side of the fence.

And protein supplements experienced little support at all in mainstream prior to about 1990. The following again reflects mainstream, peer reviewed consensus for the early 1980s :

"...protein supplements are not necessary for individuals undertaking strenuous exercise programs. Wise selection of quality protein foods will provide adequate amounts through balanced diets..."
- Williams, M.H., 1983, *Nutrition for Sport and Fitness*, WCB, Iowa, USA.

The following holds no surprises as to the attitude of mainstream nutritionists around the start of the 90's :

Protein supplements experienced little support at all in mainstream prior to about 1990.

"..Protein powders and amino acid supplements are unnecessary providing the diet is satisfactory...the saintly status of protein is dying as athletes are realizing that the steak before a strenuous event does not assist with performance...it is pointless to take extra protein...there is no need to supplement the diet with extra proteins.."
- Kilworth, L., 1990, Protein and sports performance, *Sportsmed News*, Oct 1990, p. 11-12.

And what were the physicians being taught at this time?

"...although these studies (by Lemon and others) raise intriguing questions, researchers seem to agree that most people – including athletes – are able to obtain all the protein they need through diet, without resorting to the use of supplements.."
- McCarthy, P., 1989, How much protein do athletes really need?, *Physician and Sportsmedicine*, 17(5):170-175.

Like the use of the word 'resorting'?! Gives the perception that the protein supplement user is a desperado taking some kind of addictive or health risk!

And more of the same :

"...It does not appear that protein supplements are needed to supply this 'extra' protein since athletes in general, consume adequate calories and protein..."
- Paul, G.L., 1989, Dietary protein requirements of physically active individual, *Sports Medicine, 8(3):*154-176.

And of course there was the use of 'fear' to discourage heretical behavior like breaking out of mainstream values! The old *'how long can I make the list of possibilities that rarely, if ever, have happened'* list!

"...chronic protein overloading can produce undesirable side effects....can worsen dehydration and increase the athletes risk of developing heat- related injuries...contribute to changes in renal function, total renal blood flow and glomerular filtration rate...detrimental to kidney structure and function, and increase the athlete's risk of developing renal diseases...increase the osmotic load in the intestine and produce severe gastrointestinal disturbances..."
- Wheeler, K., 1988, Proteins and amino acids, *NSCA J, 10(6):*22-29.

Fortunately not everyone went down the grim reaper path in relation to protein!

"...There does not appear to be any harm in eating excess protein in the healthy individual."
- Rozenek, R., and Stone, M.H., 1984, Protein metabolism related to athletes, *NSCA J.,* Apr-May, 42-45.

As the co-author of the above article was Michael Stone, you can see his practical experience as a lifter may have given him better insight than some other non-practitioner researchers.

But as an average *'I go to the gym and lift weights to get big and strong'* type of person, there was some sense in amongst the trash around this era – Jerry Branium (Branium, 1990, How much protein do you really need?, *Muscle and Fitness, 51(5):*105-110) asked the question in the title of an article *'How* *much protein do you really need?'*, and the sub-title is sight for sore eyes!

"Scientists argue, but bodybuilders know better!"

No wonder, they had protein-whiz researcher Peter Lemon on their advisory team!

Eating to Recover

The role of nutrition on recovery has come a long way. The work in the '80s that was arguably commercially driven to support the role of carbohydrate intake post-training to accelerate recovery probably did a lot more good than the general over-emphasis on carbohydrates that has colored the recommendations of mainstream nutritionists over the last few decades.

Bottom line – consume some type of nutrition IMMEDIATELY after training.

Having liquid nutrition straight after a workout is nothing new to those in the 'Iron Game' (the name given to the more hard core pursuit of strength training). Read some *Ironman* magazines from decades ago to see this! The scientists of the 80's wanted us all to stop that terrible, money wasting, kidney stone-creating habit! Until at least they could be seen to be one the ones who came up with the idea!

Here are my thoughts :

- Bottom line – consume some type of nutrition IMMEDIATELY after training. You will read varied times for this window of opportunity, but I suggest within the first ten to fifteen minutes. Even if for no other reason than to make sure you prioritize it and don't forget it!
- Failure to do so will allow more catabolism (muscle tissue damage) to occur. In fact, the mere delaying of this intake may increase the damage (or more accurately, miss the opportunity to negate it).

- Preferably liquid, as it may get into the bloodstream faster.
- Whether it is carbs or protein or a mix will depend on what you took in during the workout, and what you had in the two hours leading up to the workout.
- If you consumed carbs in liquid form during the workout, I lean towards a protein dominant drink. If you had water or similar with no macro-nutrients, I would consider a liquid carb intake first followed within 30 minutes by a protein dominant liquid intake or a meal.
- No matter what, look for that meal within 30-60 minutes of the workout.
- This will be influenced by your overall nutritional plan.
- As for what type of carbs or what type of proteins, I will leave that to you to decide, based on whoever is influencing you.

Possibly the most important hormones to discuss would be testosterone, cortisol and insulin.

Eating to Manipulate Hormones

The appreciation of the role of hormones and the ability of food to influence hormone release has been one of the conceptual breakthroughs in my career. This information has been bounced around by decades, but only more recently validated by mainstream science. I remember sitting in a meeting in about 1989 which included one of the more prominent and active US sport scientists, whose specialty includes this area. An article came up for discussion that I had written just prior to that meeting, and in that article I had made mention of and appreciation for the works of another scientist in the area of training, nutrition and hormone release. The scientist present was quick to criticize my reference to this other scientist and that particular work because those concepts has not been published in more reputable journals. The author I was crediting had the (shock and horror!) audacity to be sharing his concepts in the non-scientific publication know as *Powerlifting USA….*

Possibly the most important hormones to discuss would be testosterone, cortisol and insulin. All of these are big players in *Get Buffed!*™ type training. In brief, strength training can raise testosterone, which is good, but the hormone that dominates as a result of training is cortisol, which is not good. The aim is your post training nutritional strategy should be to minimize the damage caused by the cortisol, and reduce the amount and duration of the release of this hormone. Insulin is needed to transport energy into the muscle cell, but if you allow excessive release or spikes and dips in the release, you can cause problems – of particular concern for your bigger, strong and leaner goals – increased body fat. That's a very simple overview!

Nutrition Options – Volume and Type

Your body may have lost its ability to respond optimally to high volume food intake.

I believe nutrition is similar to training in that if you keep doing the same thing, the body's response slows and then halts. The solution is to vary the diet. I see two main options in varying nutrition for getting bigger, stronger and or leaner. They include :

- o Vary the volume
- o Vary the macro-nutrients

Vary the volume

This is the simplest of the two options, and the one I believe that most people should use throughout their lives. It's simple, and relatively easy. No matter whether your goal is to specifically get bigger, stronger, or leaner – this applies. Let's use the example of getting bigger. You may eat more volume (in calories). Initially this may have a positive effect. But then this may slow down. You may even notice your body fat rising as the only response after a while. Your body may have lost its ability to respond optimally to high volume food intake (or perhaps the type of food, but I will discuss that next). If you were to expose the body to a period of lower volume of food, it may then respond more positively the next time you go back to high volume eating.

Some of the variables may be how long do you eat high volume for, and how long do you eat low volume. What constitutes high volume and what low? Here is a simple yet effective combination I use for those looking to gain size/weight :

Strength Training days   : Mon, Tues, Thurs, Friday = normal
                                         (high) volume

Non-strength training days : Wed, Sat = lower volume

Recovery day   : either very low volume or higher
                                         volume

Training weeks   : 5-7 intakes per day (high volume)

Non-training weeks   : 3-4 intakes per day (lower volume)

As you can see, volume of food intake can be varied through size per meal as well as number of meals. The above is simple, yet effective. More importantly, it doesn't take too much thought or preparation, and therefore has great long-term application.

Vary the macro-nutrients

This option is perhaps more powerful, but takes more planning and thought. Since the awareness of high-fat or protein with low carbohydrate diets has been raised, this option is more acceptable. Even the mainstream are slowly becoming aware that the over-emphasis on carbohydrates through the 1980s and 90s was killing us – literally!

In the 1980s I was considered a heretic by saying that the focus on carbs and more carbs was off-track, an overemphasis. That the athletes were getting enough carbs. And that they needed to be focusing on getting more protein, not more carbs! Now we also know that the aversion to dietary fat that accompanied the high carb era was also off track!

My goal here is not to tell you which macro-nutrient you should dominate with. I don't believe in one diet fits all, all the time! What I am saying is that your next improvements may be as close as your willingness to vary your macro-nutrients. This means doing some homework, and giving up emotional attachments to some foods for at least a short period of time!

Your next improvements may be as close as your willingness to vary your macro-nutrients.

Perhaps the most popular technique is to lower carbs. This can be very effective in shifting your dominant metabolism to fat instead of carbs, but don't go overboard in extent or duration – carbs have their place!

Any reference to nutritional supplements in the below is not intended to be exclusive. That means if I didn't mention a particular supplement, don't assume I don't use or endorse it. I do mention the most dominant one however.

No single technique is best always or forever!

Eating to Get Bigger

This is where the real fun is! It is so much easier to eat for size than to eat to get lean! Here are some general guidelines :

- You need to eat every 2-3 hours!
- You should have protein in every meal.

- Aim for a total protein intake of about 1.5-3 grams per kilo of bodyweight.
- Where you sit on this range will be determined by how effective you find high protein diets for your size and weight gain.
- Because the volume is high, you can and should keep the fiber low. It won't really be low, but if you focus on high fiber foods you will have trouble eating the volume needed.
- If you are lean or young, you can afford to eat more. In some cases, especially if you are young – you should be eating ridiculously large amounts! This is one of the reasons young teenage males don't gain the weight that some of them are pursing – they are not eating enough! This is assuming they are very active. I am not referring to the young teenagers who have sedentary lifestyles and have already developed the body fat of most American adults!
- In eating programs where you are force feeding, including the examples of the highly active young teenage males, be prepared to experience the discomfort of doing so! You MUST eat, irrespective of whether you are hungry!
- Having said that, a serious loss of appetite can also be an indication that your are suffering over-training symptoms.
- If you are at the upper limit of body fat that you want, you cannot afford to eat like this. You need to be more selective, smarter. I would still recommend the above meal frequency, but you need to keep the volume per meal lower and the macro-nutrient selection becomes more of an issue.
- Never train hungry!
- Avoid stimulants and metabolism enhancers including caffeine.
- You should be using a protein supplement or similar, such as Biotest's *Grow*. The type of protein and macro-nutrient breakdown of the one you select may be

If you are lean or young, you can afford to eat more. In some cases, especially if you are young – you should be eating ridiculously large amounts!

influenced by your body fat levels and response to them.

- Creatine is a must! But cycle it. Refer to the original *Get Buffed!*™ for guidance in cycling your creatine supplementation.

Eating to Get Stronger

This has a lot of overlap with eating to get bigger, except where you don't want to gain size or total body weight. This requires a more frugal approach to volume. Over and above the guidelines listed for getting bigger, consider these additional points :

- Neural adaptations are limited by neural fatigue, which is believed to take longer to recover than metabolic fatigue.
- So look for foods and supplements that will enhance neural recovery. This includes any foods that calm or relax the body.
- Supplements considered effective for combating neural fatigue may include St. John's Wort.
- Look also for foods and supplements to contribute to your ability to neurally arouse or fire at higher levels during training. These may include some forms of uppers, such as the old *Ultimate Orange* by Champion Nutrition, or *Power*, Biotest's neurotransmitter formula containing tyrosine, DMAE and Ginkgo Biloba.
- As for foods, you need to find the optimum nutrition condition that contributes to 'feeling good' which is important for neuro-muscular strength training. I find sipping a carb solution during training powerful.
- Consider creatine, provided it doesn't throw your weight up if you are in a relative strength sport (a situation where you don't want to get heavier).
- Review the over-the-counter testosterone mimickers, such as Biotest's *Tribex*, provided they don't contraindicate any medical condition you have or

Neural adaptations are limited by neural fatigue, which is believed to take longer to recover than metabolic fatigue.

contravene any regulations you may be bound to if participating in a drug-tested sport or employment situation.

Eating to Get Leaner

There are many ways you can manipulate your eating to get leaner. I aim to focus on a few of the more powerful techniques. They are not absolutes. By this I mean sometimes you should use them, sometimes you should do it differently.

Some foods trigger more insulin release than others. You can use the Gylcemic Index or the Insulin Index to determine which foods will more likely spike insulin.

- Meal timing – never get so hungry that by the time you get to eat, you over-eat
- Don't miss meals early in the day.
- Control your insulin release - insulin release is raised when glycogen is increased in the body.
- You want a constant low level release of insulin rather than extreme highs and lows.
- Some foods trigger more insulin release than others. You can use the Gylcemic Index (GI) or the Insulin Index to determine which foods will more likely spike insulin release and which ones will provide a lower level, more constant release - the latter being more desirable most of the time. For example, the higher the food is on the GI scale, the more likely they are to trigger insulin release. For a simple division, you can consider foods with a GI rating of in excess of 70 high and those with GI rating of less than 70 low. You can also create three divisions : high, medium or low. Again, you will see many varied interpretations of this but you can work with something like : low=<60; medium=60-85; and high=>85. You should be able to find the GI index and examples of various foods in most nutritional books.
- Fiber and fat in the meal and digestive system will slow the release of insulin.
- Eat equal amounts throughout the day or slowly taper the volume as the day progresses.

- Avoid simple (high glycemic) carbs late in the day.
- Reduce your carb intake later in the day.
- Avoid eating for the 3-4 hours before you go to bed.
- Keep your water up!
- Use selected dietary and supplement fat to contribute to lowering your body fat.
- Use metabolism enhancing supplements sparingly if at all. They don't come free – they all have a downside. They will also reduce their effectiveness fairly quickly, and some can be addictive.
- If you do use them, go with more natural than chemical ones e.g. herbs such as guarana. But realize when you use herbs the potency is less controllable. This may only be an issue if you go with a poor quality brand, or are competing in a sport that has a limit or ban on caffeine.

The Forgotten Nutrients

There are certain foods and food supplements that are perhaps not considered as sexy or as marketable. Or perhaps they just don't excite people enough. I know it isn't their lack of contribution that lowers their profile, because they are major contributors! They include :

There are certain foods and food supplements that are perhaps not considered as sexy or as marketable. Or perhaps they just don't excite people enough.

- o Water
- o Fiber
- o Vitamins and Minerals

Water

If you were aware of the potential power of water, you would not neglect it! Not only is it imperative for health, it may also be anabolic, improve your strength and aid in fat loss. Now I have your interest!

From a size perspective, muscle growth will be influenced by the status of the muscle cell. Protein synthesis is affected by cellular hydration. The more hydrated the cell, the more anabolism, and vice versa. Admittedly, simply drinking more water doesn't guarantee it gets into the muscle cell. The movement of fluid into the intracellular area is more complex than that. However, in a hydrated state, your chances of cell hydration may be even less.

From a strength perspective, increased cell hydration has a leverage effect. The fuller the cell, the stronger you are. Whilst this is transient or temporary, the heavier you lift, the greater the training effect. The training effect is more permanent than the moment of training. This is one of the reasons that creatine may be effective in strength and size training – by increasing the fluid volume of the muscle cell, allowing greater strength expression.

Water may also be anabolic, improve your strength and aid in fat loss.

From a fat loss perspective, water can act as an appetite suppressant. Your hunger pains can be satisfied by water. When on a low calorie eating plan, I believe the sipping of water is even more critical to suppress these pains. There is nothing worse than being tortured by hunger pain! It can make the temptation of food harder to resist! Additionally there is evidence to suggest that water can enhance fat burning as an energy source, and glycogen sparing as side-effect.

From a health perspective, keep in mind that a higher protein or carb diet may require a higher water intake to manage the waste by-product of metabolism e.g. urea and ketones.

You can lose an average of two liters per day through normal activity. Intense training can take that up to two liters per hour. You can see that your fluid replacement needs are high and varied. You will get some of this from your food. But you will need to supplement this with water!

Fiber

Over and above the health implications of lacking fiber in the diet (e.g. bowel complications), fiber plays an important nutritional role in getting bigger, stronger and or leaner. An absence or the reduction of fiber in the diet can result in less control of the insulin response, and a failure to benefit from the thermogenic cost of digesting the food.

To illustrate this, lets review fruit juice as opposed to eating the whole fruit. It is fruit minus the fiber. The absence of the fiber means that it will spike your insulin faster, and that it loses the thermogenic effect that the original food would have that is lacking in the juice. Fruit juice becomes a poorer option.

Vitamins and Minerals

Fiber plays an important nutritional role in getting bigger, stronger and or leaner.

It is rare that you find an article on vitamins and minerals in modern day bodybuilding magazines. In fact, this domain is left mainly to the health industry. There was a time when this wasn't the case. In the late 1970s American strength coach Bill Starr wrote a classic book titled *The Strongest Shall Survive*. In that book he dedicated pages to the discussion of vitamins and minerals. The recommendations he made all those years ago have stood the test of time, including research support for his specific doses.

Interestingly, Fred Hatfield gave to similar conclusions in writing his book *Bodybuilding – A Scientific Approach* in the mid 1980s. In fact, if you want to check out how ahead of this time Starr was, compare his 1979 recommendations to the average of four current day medical/scientific experts (Drs. Passwater, Colgan, Murray and Strand) as presented by Lyle MacWilliam 2001 book *Comparative Guide to Nutritional Supplements*. Published 22 years later! Keeping in mind that Starr's recommendations were for *"athletes who are spending 2-4 hours of physical training each day. If the athlete is not participating (in training)...then his nutritional needs will be much lower"*, and that the average of four experts provided by MacWilliam is for the average person (who you can assume is not training intensely if at all) – you gain an appreciation of how far ahead of their time some of the guidelines provided by leaders in the Iron Game have been!

Bottom line is – if you take a vitamin/mineral supplement based on the RDA (recommend dietary allowances) or RDI (recommended dietary intake) levels – you are probably wasting your time. But if you take a high dose vitamin/mineral supplement, based on information so old that even science as validated it (!), you will notice a short term and long term difference!

If you take a vitamin / mineral supplement based on the RDA levels – you are probably wasting your time.

So why the lack of focus on them nowadays? I suspect it's an extension of the need for instant gratification. People feel that a multi-vitamin/mineral supplement is not going to make them big and strong within six weeks so why bother. I take a different approach. I believe they should be the first supplement you add, and the last one you delete. I question the ability of your body to optimally digest and utilize your other performance enhancing supplements in the presence of inadequate vitamins and minerals in the diet. And if you believe that even with high volume nutrition you are going to achieve your vitamin and mineral targets, we are probably looking at different targets!

Another reason I suspect for the lack of focus on these basic building blocks, vitamins and minerals, is that the majority of the vitamin/mineral supplements produced are so low dose, so inconstantly dosed, and so poorly manufactured, that no-one gets any long term benefits let alone short term benefits.

After over two decades of experimenting with vitamins I have discovered adequate evidence for the dosages I was let to believe were needed from reading Starr's work over twenty years. Perhaps one of the best books on this subject is Lyle MacWilliam's *Comparative Guide to Nutritional Supplements*.

If you found a vitamin and mineral supplement that gave you more energy, reduced recovery time from training, better protection from free radicals, better sleep – would you show more interest? I thought so! It does exist. You can learn more at www.unitoday.net/king. Athletes that I have worked with over the last few years have had fantastic response to this brand.

If you found a vitamin and mineral supplement that gave you more energy, reduced recovery time from training, better protection from free radicals, better sleep – would you show more interest?

Chapter 5
Goal Setting and Measuring
Giving you direction and feedback!

As you get more advanced in your training, you may experience the law of diminishing returns. In essence, your rate of change slows. You will find you need to get smarter about your training to get the results you want.

One technique is to exploit the power of goal setting and measuring. Simply implementing these techniques is virtually guaranteed to give you results!

In *Get Buffed!*™ the original book, I discussed guidelines for goal setting and measuring. What I want to do in this book is to go further in this area. I am going to present symmetry models. The power of this is it gives you comparisons or yardsticks by which to compare your shape and progress with. This can be motivating, educating, and provide direction. If you are wondering why I don't give strength guidelines e.g. how much should you be able to bench relative to your shoulder press etc. I find them fraught with error and misinterpretation. They may look or sound great but I believe they are inaccurate and misleading. They have some application for say a competitive weight lifter or powerlifter, but their value stops there.

It gives you comparisons or yardsticks by which to compare your shape and progress.

The areas I will address in this chapter include :

- ❏ Symmetry guides
- ❏ Somatotypes
- ❏ Recording your workout

Symmetry Guides

The three symmetry guides I will share with you include :

- ○ The Body Measurements
- ○ The Extremity Measurements
- ○ The Willougby Symmetrometer

The overall aim and benefit of these guides is to provide or encourage symmetry in physiques. Without some guidance it's easy to develop relative imbalances in appearance.

The overall aim and benefit of these guides is to provide or encourage symmetry in physiques. Without some guidance it's easy to develop relative imbalances in appearance.

The Body Measurements

These are age-old figures passed down through the years in strength training circles and they go like this – your thigh measurement should be about 10" smaller than your waist measurement, which should be about 10" smaller than your chest measurement.

For example, you may have or aim for :

Chest	: 45 "
Waist	: 35 "
Upper Thigh	: 25"

These are only rough guidelines but I found them valuable. I believe they came from a time when a lifter would train with a balance of the powerlifts, the Olympic lifts, and general bodybuilding movements.

The Extremity Measurements

These are relevant to the circumferences of the lower legs, upper arm and neck. It goes like this : your calf measurement should be about the same size as your upper arm (flexed) and your neck measurements (taken above the Adam's Apple).

For example, you may have or aim for :

Calf	:	17"
Upper arm	:	17"
Neck	:	17"

Again, these are only rough guidelines but provide direction and food for thought.

The Willougby Symmetrometer

This is a fantastic tool that I found in Phillip Rasch's book *Weight Training* first published in 1966 and again in 1975. He presented a table in this book, that he credited to David Willougby, an American scientist. Willougby is described by Rasch as *"an anthropometrist and historian of weight training"*.

This table allows you to plot your circumferences for your neck, upper arm, lower arm, wrist, chest, waist, hips, upper legs, lower legs and ankles – as well as your height and weight. Ideally, this line would be vertical. Any deviations to the right or left would suggest over or under developed muscles. This table was developed by the David Willougby and based on his extensive years of observation, measurement and study of well-developed athletes and bodybuilders. It was designed to allow any individual (male) to measure his body and compare it to this chart for feedback on his symmetry.

Despite the passing of time since this information was collated, it was good enough for me during the peak of my serious strength training years, and I believe it would still be

These are only rough guidelines but provide direction and food for thought.

good enough for anyone in this day or the future who seeks feedback on their progress towards developing a symmetrical physique.

Rasch also presented the circumference measurements for each of the AAU Mr. Americas from 1940-1974, which he admitted needed to be considered in the light of likely exaggeration. Never-the-less, this table also makes interesting reading!

Somatotypes

Recording your training is not hip, and is not supported in the majority of marketing so you may wonder why I stress it so much.

I wanted to make a brief comment in relation to body or somatotyping. I am referring to the categorization of body types into ectomorph (tall and skinny), endomorphs (short and carrying more body fat), and mesomorphs (stocky or muscular build). I am not a big fan of this technique. I don't care what you started with. Provided you don't limit your potential with limiting beliefs, you can develop any physique you want!

Recording Your Workout

I believe that at this level, recording of training is mandatory. I have no time for those who don't record their training, and yet expect to achieve high levels. Perhaps in the presence of drugs this is possible, but irrespective to your decisions in this regard – you should record.

One of my favorite quotes in this area is by the West German strength researcher Dr. Dietmar Schmidtbleicher, who wrote :

"Regardless of the training method practiced, the coach as well as the athlete must precisely record the number of training units, the intensity, the number of reps, the rest interval, so that the training goal can be precisely established."

I have training diaries for the last twenty years plus. I experienced great gains in my training history and I give some of this credit to the fact that I recorded my training. Recording your training supports recording and setting your goals.

I understand that recording your training is not hip, and is not supported in the majority of marketing so you may wonder why I stress it so much. I am not teaching you what marketing trends would have you believe. I am teaching you what I believe you should do to achieve your goals!

A good training diary will have provision to record :

- Planning of Training
- Strength Training
- Speed Training
- Endurance Training
- Flexibility Training
- Nutrition

You can use a commercially prepared diary such as the Get Buffed! ™ Training Diary, or you can simply buy a blank notebooks from your local store.

You can use a commercially prepared diary such as the *Get Buffed!*™ Training Diary, or you can simply buy a blank notebook from your local store. Make sure it has a strong side bind so it doesn't fall apart too quickly!

Information I recommend that you should record on your strength training days will include the information listed in the example recording sheet on the following page.

Recommended Reference Material

The *Get Buffed!*™ **Training Diary** – available at www.getbuffed.net

Stage No : _____ Week No. : _____ Day : _____

Date : _____ Venue : _____ Bodyweight : _____

Start warm-up Time : _____ Start Workout Time : _____

End Workout Time : _____ Total Workout Time : _____

Pre-workout comments : _____

Exercise	1		2		3		4		Rest
	W	R	W	R	W	R	W	R	Period
Warm-Up Notes									

Post workout comments :

_____

_____

_____

_____

Chapter 6

The Psychology of Getting Buffed!™

Training the mind!

What I want to share with you in this chapter is what I believe to be very powerful. It has the potential to make a big difference on the outcome. What I will share with you is practical ideas and concepts that you can apply easily and immediately.

These include :

- ❑ The Psychology of Getting Bigger, Stronger and Leaner
- ❑ The Psychology of Recovery
- ❑ The Psychology of Lifting
- ❑ The Psychology of Load vs. Technique

What I am going to teach you is the power of being the person who would do the things that would result in achieving the goal. To become the person you want to be in the mind firstly. And to adopt the positive attitude of appreciation of what you have yet dissatisfaction with the level that it is at, enough to take massive action!

You may be surprised to know I place as much if not more importance on the psychology of these goals than training and nutrition.

You may be surprised to know I place as much if not more importance on the psychology of these goals than training and nutrition. Quite simply I respect and endorse the belief that the mind is more powerful than the body. That the body creates, allows or disallows the physical result. Therefore the power of training and nutrition is undermined or dwarfed by the power of the mind. You can train and eat to get a certain result yet your success or failure will, in my mind have been influenced more by the conscious and sub-conscious decisions you make than the training or diet.

It's so great to be able to share these concepts with you. When I write or present in most short duration mediums, I give more shallow content, to some extent what most people want to hear. I appreciate that for example a magazine may not enhance it's sales if I was published writing about something so abstract as psychology. Much of this medium is pandering to the instant gratification needs of the reader. Who as a result need a new instant gratification idea each subsequent issue!

What I am teaching you is that the mindset is more powerful than the action itself, and the result will be greater when the mindset and the action are congruent!

There is a common belief in society that all one needs is to know what to do. What I am teaching you is that the mindset is more powerful than the action itself, and the result will be greater when the mindset and the action are congruent!

The Psychology of Getting Bigger, Stronger and Leaner

Within this discussion I will address :

- o Your Environment
- o Body fat and Washboards
- o Colors
- o Clothing
- o Eating Equipment
- o Eating
- o Not Training

- Feelings about the Pump and Muscle Soreness
- Measuring
- Associations

Your Environment

When training to get bigger, I want you to create the mentality of the USA state of Texas – BIG! Everything becomes BIG. You think BIG. You relate to BIG. Your goal should be to look BIG in clothes, not relying on being stripped to the waist for someone to realize you lift. Surround yourself with samples of those who have achieved more than you. This is where the bodybuilding and strength magazine come in handy!

When training to get stronger, surround yourself with examples of strength. If you don't already do so, subscribe to true strength publications, such as *Powerlifting USA, International Weightlifting, Milo* and so on. Spend time with stronger people, and people who also value this result.

When training to get bigger, I want you to create the mentality of the USA state of Texas – BIG!

When training to get lean, surround yourself with examples of leanness. Spend time with leaner people, and people who reward this condition. Get exposed to those who can help you create the mindset of leanness. For example, psychologist and personal development expert Denis Waitley has an audio tape set titled *The Psychology of Living LEAN'*.

Body Fat and Washboards

When I hear about someone who says that are trying to get bigger but it isn't happening, I do what I call a trouble shoot. I run through all the training and nutritional variables looking for a flaw, a way to improve. I don't get surprised when I don't see one. Or more accurately when the person fails to verbalize one! They just can't understand why they cannot get bigger!

I then dig deeper and invariably I find a subconscious belief or value that is not congruent with getting bigger. A value or belief they have a greater emotional attachment to than their expressed goal of getting bigger.

One of these most common counter-productive attachments is their true, deep down fear of loosing their low body fat appearance. You would be surprised at how many people possess this fear! It initially became apparent to me when dealing with former track sprinters who had turned professional football player. They just 'couldn't put on weight'! I learnt that deep down they just didn't want to loose their *Men's Health* 'front cover' looks'!

Get this clear – putting on a bit of body fat whilst pursing gaining size is OK! And likely! No, I am not saying you have to turn into a beach ball. Just loose that fixation with having super-low body fat and washboard abs!

Unless you are a strength athlete competing in weight divisions or relative strength sports, don't get fixated with low body fat. That attitude only gets in the way! I am not suggesting you can or should blow out. Just make sure that you are not allowing a leanness focus to limit your strength gains.

A totally different attitude is needed for those pursing leanness – you need to focus and take pride in this body part! It will be your ultimate assessment. With males in particular, this can be the site of your greatest fat deposition.

Colors

According to author Patrick Ellis in his book titled *Who Dares Sells*, "*...colors are closely linked to emotions. When someone uses a particular color or a preference of colors in the home or office, or in clothing, jewelry, personal effects or footwear, they are letting you know something non-verbally. In fact, the deliberate choice of colors reveals how the person views themselves.*"

One of these most common counter-productive attachments is their true, deep down fear of loosing their low body fat appearance.

How do you view yourself? BIG! Or Strong, or Lean!

Ellis sites a Dr. J.R. Wurtman of the Massachusetts Institute of Technology in Boston who claimed that after food, light is the next most important influence on our bodily functions, because *"…color affects us at a deep psychological level and the electro-magnetic energy of color has far-reaching effects on the endocrine system."*

Blue is one of my favorite colors to achieve the relaxed environment I believe important to accelerate recovery. According to Ellis, blue is *"relaxing and gives a feeling of space and calm, diminishing excitability and urgency."* What do we want to do when we are not training? Relax!!

Those pursuing lower body fat may associate with or benefit from being exposed to brighter colors. Just an idea!

Clothing

For those pursing BIG, when you buy clothes, get them loose. You will be growing into them. When you buy clothes be conscious that you will be growing out of them soon. Be prepared to have a variety of sizes of the same clothing item in the wardrobe!

One of the great things about wearing bigger clothes is that it encourages you to have a strong and burning desire to grow into them!

One of the great things about wearing bigger clothes is that it encourages you to have a strong and burning desire to grow into them! On the other hand, if you wear your little brothers shirt (something tight) you are likely to conclude you are SO big and lack desire to get bigger!

When it comes to training clothes, I am strongly against less clothing than a t-shirt. Now I know that sounds strange but hear me out. I feel that you need to have a desire to look big in clothes, not needing to strip to realize your size.

Those who show more flesh can easily conclude they are big enough. I want that powerful degree of dissatisfaction. There is a significant psychological distinction between seeing your muscles contraction and temporarily pumped (and associating that with you have already arrived!) and the psychology of not seeing the result until it is extremely obvious from under a t-shirt!

The way someone dresses tells me so much about that person. I believe people wear their brothers shirts for one of two main reasons – they are either insecure and want the positive attention. Or they really believe they are massive.

To me, a truly massive person doesn't need to wear a T-back singlet to get the message across!

Now for clothing colors – over and above your skin and hair color, I believe that relaxing colors and styles should dominate your selection. Body language and personality type analysts read 'comfortable with one's body' into loosely fitting clothes. There is a perception that this person is in touch with their bodies. This is more critical outside the gym than in

Those pursing Lean may take a totally different approach. They may want to see the rewards, show more mid-section, show more of the taper from the shoulders to the waist that having lower body fat allows to be seen.

Eating Equipment

For those aiming for BIG, you are probably going to eating large amounts of food. Get big eating equipment! Get a BIG cup, a BIG plate, and a BIG bowl. Just surround yourself with BIG!

The added benefit is if you are struggling to complete your meals. A big serving on a bigger plate looks small!

Get BIG eating equipment! Get a BIG cup, a BIG plate, and a BIG bowl. Just surround yourself with BIG!

Additionally, people in your inner circle get the message and start treating you like a BIG kind of person! Applying the sociology theory of 'Cooley's looking glass self' (we see ourselves through the eyes of others), we further gain the reinforcement that we are BIG!

When David J. Schwartz wrote the great self-development book *The Magic of Thinking* book, he didn't use lower case on the letters 'Big' on the front cover – he made them BIG!

Now in colors again, there are some really relaxing colors you can get on cups, plates and bowls. Selecting colors that would be in place in a Hawaiian resort would be a safe starting point!

The reverse can be said for those on a restricted food intake. If you use a smaller plate, your smaller size portion can look bigger and help you feel better about the smaller portion! It also means physically you are limited to how much food you can put on your plate!

Eating

Those pursing BIG need to learn to love food! For most men, that's pretty easy! Live your life around food. Set your clock or a countdown timer to go off to make sure you are not so much as minutes late for this meal! Eat your food slowly, in a relaxed environment.

Alternatively, those focusing on getting Lean may want to show appreciation for food, but not allow such a fixation as above.

Not Training

Do not equate taking a day off training with getting smaller. When I find people who have this perception, they invariably chronically over-train and never reach their potential. Focus

Do not equate taking a day off training with getting smaller. When I find people who have this perception, they invariably chronically over-train and never reach their potential.

on the benefits of recovery. See yourself growing as your body recovers!

Do not equate taking a day off training with getting fatter. I have seen very sad physiques on those who fall into this psychological trap. More training will not equate to a better physique! It may mean less total body weight, but I doubt you wanted to lose a lot of muscle also!

Feelings about the Pump and Muscle Soreness

Whilst I believe that muscle soreness and the 'pump' feeling have some relationship or correlation with an optimal training state, don't see them as exclusive. If you equate training entirely with these feelings, you will over-train. And be conscious not to kill the goose that laid the golden eggs. Don't train for the 'pump'. Instead, use it as a guide to when to stop training. So many times I see extra sets performed in a hope to regain or retain the pump, or to experience more muscle soreness in the belief that the more that these feelings are experienced, the better! Not true! Hey, I may have even made that mistake many times before as well! Okay, not maybe – I have! As no doubt you have no! Learn from your mistakes!

Set the frequency of testing for time periods that allow reasonable time to see a change. For example, don't take your body fat daily, or even weekly (except in extreme 'cutting' situations).

Measuring

Whilst measuring is important (e.g. bodyweight, circumferences, etc.) realize that they are indirect measures. That means they also come with a degree of error. Don't jump off the closest bridge when they don't give you what you wanted to see. Conversely, if there is a pattern of inadequate results, don't ignore that. Finally, set the frequency of testing for time periods that allow reasonable time to see a change. For example, don't take your body fat daily, or even weekly (except in extreme 'cutting' situations). Generally speaking, monthly or every second week would be more accurate and place you under less pressure.

Associations

Associate with people who share your goals but ideally have achieved them to a higher level. For example, if you are pursuing BIG hang with bigger people. Train with them. Don't go looking for smaller people. Find someone who is prepared to let a smaller person train with and learn from them. You will find some are more concerned about holding you back so you don't get bigger than them! Avoid them!

The Psychology of Recovery

I find it interesting the reluctance people have to take rest days or rest weeks. Once you appreciate the physiological reality that any loss if any you experience from a rest day or week is quickly reversed and then you are rewarded even further with gains, you ideally will use them. But I am aware of the psychological component of this reluctance – fear and anxiety. The image in your head that missing so much as one workout will result in your body deflating like a blow up doll stuck with the wrong pin...

Learn to make your decisions about training with your rational side and not your emotional side! This is why having a coach with this ability is so good!

Get over it! Learn to make your decisions about training with your rational side and not your emotional side! This is why having a coach with this ability is so good! Allows the athlete to drive their training through their emotions, and another person to make rational decisions based on the emotional response of the athlete to training.

I also have come upon many individuals striving to enhance their physique or strength through weight training, who fail to (or chose to ignore) the limited impact their excessively busy and or stressful lifestyle/work have on the training effect. To optimize the training effect from strength training, you must be prepared to alter your lifestyle and or work to support this, including a slower pace and more recovery activity. If you feel you cannot (or are unwilling to) alter your lifestyle or work (and I appreciate that as you get further along in life other things take greater priority) then alter your training to suit this standard of recovery! And don't complain about your less than optimal gains! It's simply a trade-off. The more your life revolves around the training process (which includes recovery) the better the result that you will get!

The Psychology of Lifting

Perhaps the most important issues I can address in advance for this phase is the concept of arousal. Maximal load lifting is as much about the psychology as it is about the physiology. If you get under a maximum or near maximum load with a low focus and low level of arousal, in most cases you will get buried. There may be some rare individuals who are exceptions to this, but chances are you will benefit from learning techniques to ensure the level of arousal meets the demands of the load.

Now I am not talking about the jokes that scream and carry-on, look around the gym to count how many people are watching, and then proceed to do another 13 reps! Having said that, if the arousal technique you have mastered is a noisy one that's okay. This is not about noise pollution. This is about whether the technique you use is for show or go. Obviously, I like the ones that are functional....

Now I am going to give you some tips on how to match your level of arousal to the load. I am not saying you need to use any or all of them. But it may provide some guidance for those who recognize that this is an area they could improve on. What I am sharing with you is not out of a sports psychology textbook, but rather methods I have observed and used personally and professionally.

- o Visualization
- o Imagery
- o Body temperature

o   Rest period length and content

o   Re-focusing after the rest period

Visualization

There is a concept in lifting that the outcome of a set is determined before it is begun. What is meant here is the state of mind that exists immediately prior to the set may have a huge bearing on the outcome. If you are thinking, *"I hope I can get this"* you probably won't. If you are wondering, *"I wonder if the spotters are going to be quick enough?"* they will probably be needed. But if you are thinking about how you are going to SUCCESSFULLY complete the set or rep, running this through your mind in a positive and determined manner, you will probably do just that!

Now this mind state has to be very strong and firm. If there is any weakening of this resolve, even just for a second, in the lead up to the set, you may be gone!

Most heavy lifting in gymnasiums is done on the basis of wishful thinking. At least this is my observation. I suspect that many load the bar up beyond their expectation of themselves, knowing they will fail, but happy in the thought of what an impact it will make when people see the amount of weight on the bar (forget about the minor detail of whether you can lift it). Consequently most bench exercises become high load upright rows for the spotter!

If you have had this pattern of behavior, you are going to have to work especially hard to adapt a new approach, an approach similar to the one I have described above!

Imagery

In addition to 'seeing' the lift being successfully completed, there are many other techniques you can use to 'get yourself up there'. One of my favorites is to picture someone who you

If you are thinking about how you are going to SUCCESSFULLY complete the set or rep, running this through your mind in a positive and determined manner, you will probably do just that!

really want to out-lift, seeing them lift a weight like this, and being driven by a strong desire to out lift them. Even though they are not likely to be in your presence, you use an image of them to provide extra motivation to exceed them. And exceeding them begins with the bar right there in front of you!

This technique of imagery is used by many competitive athletes in various sporting endeavors – so why not you too? It doesn't even have to be someone you know personally. It may not even be about the respective strength levels. It may be about a person who picture you are familiar with, and whose physical attributes you aspire to.

You just need to find a reason to do it. Your body is naturally protective, homeostatic, resisting stresses and change. You are about to go and stress it! You need to remove or elevate the natural inhibitory or protective mechanisms.

Immediately following a max strength set, walk slowly around the gym to accelerate recovery. Then sit down, and place at least a towel around your shoulders.

Body temperature

When you complete a lift and go into the rest period, your body initially elevates in function (heart rate, respiratory etc), and then lowers. Most of the rest periods you will use in maximal strength training will be between 3-5 minutes long on average. You can get pretty cold in this time. Getting cold makes it harder to attain optimal arousal, and may also have a negative impact on neuro-muscular function. So to avoid this, here is what I recommend: immediately following a maximum effort set, walk slowly around the gym to accelerate recovery. Then sit down, and place at least a towel around your shoulders. Whether you use more clothes (e.g. track pants), how big the towel should be, and how tightly you should wrap it around yourself, will all be influenced by room temperature.

Now the advantages are not just in maintaining the body temperature more suited to performance. There is an added bonus. The towel should not come off until the last thing. At this time, there will be a 'shock' effect as the room temperature and air meet the skin. At this time your body temperature, due to the use of the towel, may be higher than room temperature. So the air feels colder when the towel comes off, and this invokes the 'fight or flight' autonomic response – put simply, it jars you into action even further!

Rest period length and content

In maximal-strength strength training you will want to use a relatively long rest period. This presents a number of challenges, including managing of temperature and focus. The plan I recommend has a number of phases within the rest period. These phases are designed to manage optimally the challenges that arise from longer rest periods. They include:

- **Recover :** As I mentioned above, walk around after the set you have just done, to aid and accelerate recovery. It's not a race or a power-walk – just move at a pace you feel comfortable. I expect 30 seconds to 1 minute is adequate – this is not an aerobic session!

- **Get feedback :** Assuming you have spotters working with you (which I hope is the case!), time to get their feedback. Here's an important tip – ask them what they thought before you tell them what you thought! And don't intimidate them into saying what they think you want to hear.

- **Replenish :** Take the steps to replenish – sip from your drink bottle, another bite on that appropriate food.

- **Decide on next load :** By now you will have had time to think about the load for the next set. I hope you had a plan before you started, but I also hope you approach load selection as a flexible issue, one to be influenced by outcomes on the day. I would imagine you may need to consult your training log again, and perhaps enter in the load for the next set now. Not the reps – just the load (a little trick I use with great effectiveness!). I feel if I write the reps in before I do the

Consult your training log again, and perhaps enter in the load for next set now. Not the reps – just the load.

set, I think I have done the effort. I have to earn those reps before they get entered into my training log!

- **Prepare equipment** : This is critical – you do not want to be adjusting equipment at the last minute. Or worse still, you don't want to be going into the set with an incorrect load! Make sure rack height is good, the correct weight loaded, position of bar on racks is symmetrical etc.
- **Recuperate** : Now it's time to sit down, towel on, do nothing. Don't let the mind wander too far here, but don't get too hyped up. Relax, but stay close mentally.
- **Refocus** : Now is the time to take the arousal level back up to optimal. Allow whatever time it takes, use whatever techniques work. Towel stays on. The rest periods in Stage 4 can get very long (up to 7 minutes) so this ability to refocus is paramount).
- **Approach** : Only approach the bar once the arousal levels and focus/determination is optimal! Towel comes off in the approach; use the same direction and number of steps in the approach to the bar.

Let me make it very clear – having a focus on technique does not equate to lifting light all the time.

Now you may feel that these techniques are the exclusive domain of competitive lifter, and that they may not apply to you. Yes, competitive lifters do tend to master them. But why can't you use them also?

The Psychology of Load vs. Technique

Because I place a premium on skill execution and learning in strength exercises, a common knee jerk reaction by some is that you can only ever use light weights with my methods. Let me make it very clear – having a focus on technique does not equate to lifting light all the time. Provided the skill is mastered, load potential is unlimited.

The reality is that as anyone gets closer to their maximum at any given stage of their training career, some technical breakdown may occur. You don't drop the weight in horror – you finish the set, decide whether the technical deviation was not so bad that further reps or set cannot be done (and it rarely is in a well trained lifter) and commit that in the next general preparatory phase and subsequent buildups you take your technical limits of work capacity even higher. Again, this may be something only those with greater discipline and appreciation of the long term, bigger picture can relate to.

If technical breakdown does occur, we place special focus in the start of our subsequent multi-stage program on re-correcting the lift, and improving the load and joint angle at which technical breakdown may occur. This is a continual re-adjustment of techniques. No-one is immune from this reality.

So in the early stages of any program, prioritize and place highest value on adherence to technique, not load. Slowly shift this focus over the length of the program, so that by the end, the prioritization on load is greater than the prioritization technique. Then be prepared to return back to technical priority in the start of a subsequent program. You need emotional flexibility – don't get too attached to either!

If technical breakdown does occur, we place special focus in the start of our subsequent multi-stage program on re-correcting the lift.

Chapter 7
The Warm Up
Laying the foundations for the workout!

The warm up deserves more attention than often given. It has multiple potential benefits, but should be modified to suit your needs. The following will give you some guide as to how to manipulate the warm up to suit your needs at any given time. Note, that means that you may have a different warm up approach for different workouts within the same week, or different stages, or from program to program. It is a variable that you can and should manipulate!

In this chapter we will discuss :

- ❑ Aims and Potential Benefits of the Warm Up
- ❑ Limitations and Potential Pitfalls of the Warm Up
- ❑ Types of Warm Up
- ❑ The Relationship Between Warm Up and Different Muscle Groups
- ❑ Warm Up Guidelines
- ❑ Passive Strategies to Enhance and Support the Warm Up

You may have a different warm up approach for different workouts within the same week, or different stages, or from program to program.

Aims and Potential Benefits of Warm Up

The warm up can be used to :

- o Raise body temperature to increase neuro-muscular firing potential o Raise body temperature to reduce joint friction in specific joints

o Reduce injury potential

o Burn energy or calories / raise metabolism for the next few days

Raise body temperature to increase neuro-muscular firing potential

Your ability to recruit muscle fiber is influenced by your body temperature. This is one of the reasons that ability to express strength and the optimal time to train strength is influenced by the time of the day – early in the morning, your body temperature is low and your ability to fire the muscles is low.

Your ability to recruit muscle fiber is influenced by your body temperature. This is one of the reasons that ability to express strength and the optimal time to train strength is influenced by the time of the day.

So you can use the warm up to enhance the ability to train, and the quality of the training and therefore the training effect. Of course, more is not better – there are optimal levels in every area so review the following information for greater understanding of optimal.

Raise body temperature to reduce joint friction in specific joints

As the temperature rises in the joint, there is an elevation of the fluid levels that contribute to lubrication of the joint. This is a fantastic concept, so powerful in practical application. For those who have advanced joint wear, this can mean the difference between being able to train pain free and with pain. For those who don't have joint wear, you are the minority and must have had a very gentle life to date, or be very young! I believe that most people have joint wear that they are not even aware of. This is quite normal. This low level joint wear can, I believe, lower the ability of your muscles or inhibit them from firing to their full potential – without you even being aware of it!

So no matter what your current joint status is – there is a powerful reason to employ warm ups to raise joint temperature – to minimize or prevent further degeneration.

Reduce injury potential

This is an area that many in mainstream has sought to deny as a benefit of the warm up. Sure, performing a warm up is not a guarantee against injury. But common sense (which apparently is not common) can see that the warm up can have acute performance benefits (better muscle firing, less inhibition from joint wear or other physiological inhibitors) as well as injury prevention benefits e.g. less joint damage over time (chronic wear).

So don't underestimate the role of warm ups – be they general or specific warm up activities. I will explain the difference between general and specific warm up shortly (see Types of Warm Up).

Performing a warm up is not a guarantee against injury. But common sense can see that the warm up can have acute performance benefits as well as injury prevention benefits.

Burn energy or calories now / raise metabolism for the next few days

There is potential to use the warm up as an energy burning workout in itself. This does of course have implications for the subsequent workout, but depending on the type of workout to follow and your priorities in training, this is definitely a possibility. For example, should your priorities be such that lowering your body fat through that particular activity was a high priority and the workout to follow was short or easy and of lower priority, this would be appropriate.

For time efficiency this can be a great option, so if you are in a situation where you want to burn calories and do a strength workout within, for example, one hour – and you feel you needed a solid warm up (e.g. because you were about to do multi-joint lower body exercises) then this can be a great option.

Remember, burning calories is not just about how many you burn now, but the energy used as a result of the elevation in metabolism that can occur for hours through to days after a workout.

Limitations and Potential Pitfalls of the Warm Up

Now that you are aware of the aims and potential benefits of the warm up, don't assume that more is better, or that a warm-up is needed or beneficial in all situations. The following discusses potential limitations and pitfalls associated with or presented by the warm up.

This includes :

- o Excessive fatigue
- o Excessive heat
- o Efficient use of time
- o Potential joint aggravation

Always assess by projecting forward or anticipating the impact on the workout that may occur from the residual fatigue resulting from the warm up.

Excessive fatigue

Always assess by projecting forward or anticipating the impact on the workout that may occur from the residual fatigue resulting from the warm up. Yes, you can overdo the warm up and negatively impact the workout e.g. lose energy, have less strength. However, don't assume that just because the warm up caused fatigue, and even if that residual fatigue reduced work capacity in the workout, that it is inappropriate. Appropriateness is determined by your needs.

Generally speaking, for maximal strength workouts, and definitely towards the end of these phases when you may be pursing personal bests, avoid residual fatigue from the warm ups. However in hypertrophy phases, the residual fatigue may actually be a positive contributor!

Excessive heat

I spoke earlier of the values of elevating body temperature. But remember there could be an optimal level. Your specific goals will determine what is optimal body temperature. Excessive heat may be related to excessive fatigue and dehydration. The level of heat that is optimal will be for example related to the type of exercises or muscle groups you plan to train. The deeper the muscle group, the more you will need to warm up, recognizing that core temperature may take longer to rise than peripheral or skin temperature.

When selecting the type of warm up, remember that there is potential for joint damage from the warm up....So you need to ensure that the type, intensity and duration of the workout is consistent with your capabilities PAIN FREE.

For example, I believe that raising core temperature with a longer warm up optimizes the squat performance. However the same could not be said for a smaller, more peripheral muscle group such as the upper arm.

Efficient use of time

I always encourage a review of time efficiency. Even if for no other reason than the length of training can influence the time frame between meals! If time is no obstacle, I see support for the time between the start of the warm up and the end of the workout being as long as two hours. But not everyone has this time, and some may not have the recovery capacity for this. So when you are reducing the time frame of the total workout time, the need for efficiency becomes greater.

When condensing the time frame of each component of the workout, ensure that the relative time frames still reflect the priorities you hold at that time.

Potential joint aggravation

When selecting the type of warm up, remember that there is potential for joint damage from the warm up. In most circumstances, no activity precedes the warm up. So you need to ensure that the type, intensity and duration of the workout is consistent with your capabilities PAIN FREE.

For example, there are some conditions such as chronic knee pain that should have a light stretch before you do any loading on a stationary exercise bike. Remember, once you aggravate a joint, it is usually aggravated for that whole workout and sometimes the whole day. You don't want to aggravate a joint leading into the workout!

The specific warm up SHOULD NEVER BE DELETED! Having said that, there is no such thing as never.

Types of Warm Up

There are generally speaking two types of warm up, and they include :

- o A general warm up; and
- o A specific warm up.

General Warm Up

The general warm up is as the name suggests, less specific to the target training activity than the specific warm up. The general warm up and the specific warm up would usually both occur within the one workout, with the general warm up preceding the specific warm up. There may be situations where the general warm up is deleted (such as say an upper arm strength workout) but the specific warm up SHOULD NEVER BE DELETED!

Having said that, there is no such thing as never. I wanted to be strong in that statement simply to reinforce it should be rarely deleted, and only when accompanied by a solid rationalization e.g. a street fighter wanting to gain adaptation to fighting from a cold start. Even in these cases, it would not be the basis of long-term training, but a variation on training to gain a specific adaptation.

The aim of the general warm up is primarily to prepare the total body for training. This includes raising core temperature, lengthening out the tissues to be used in preparation, increasing the ability to recruit the target muscles, and ideally also involves raising the temperature of the joints to be trained.

This final comment indicates that even within the general warm up, your activity can be general or specific along a continuum. For example, the stationary exercise bike (of all the equipment found in the average gym) is one of the best total body general warm up activities for most people. However a rowing ergometer, which may have similar impact on elevating total body temperature, may not have the specific preparation of the knee joint as does the stationary bike – and therefore the stationary bike prior to a leg workout could be considered a more appropriate (due to specificity) general warm up activity than the rower.

The stationary exercise bike is one of the best total body general warm up activities for most people.

Therefore, a general warm up may consist of :

- A body temperature raising activity.
- A stretching activity.
- Drills aimed to improve target muscle contraction. I call these 'control drills'.

Specific Warm Up

A specific warm up has many benefits. It should ensure elevation of the target joints and muscles. It should provide rehearsal of the movement, for skill rehearsal. It should provide progressive exposure to loading. It should allow confirmation that the equipment is positioned and set up appropriately, rather than finding out anything untoward during the work sets.

What we call warm up sets in strength training are the specific warm up sets. These specific warm up sets should ideally be performed :
- With the exact body position to be used in the work set.
- On the same equipment that is to be used in the workout.
- In a progressive exposure to more loading through a series of sets.

Warm up set protocols are discussed in the original *Get Buffed!*™ book.

The Relationship Between Warm Up and Different Muscle Groups

I lean towards the stationary bike because it does the job without being too demanding, but am open to any activity based on your needs and situation.

Generally speaking, the following will influence the type of general warm up I recommend :

- Size of muscle group to be training.
- Number of joints involved in the type of exercises to be used.

This is pretty straight-forward : if the workout is going to involve big muscle groups using multi-joint type exercises, I will use more extensive general warm ups. In contrast, if the workout is going to be small muscles groups, and or including single joint exercises, I may go so far as to forgo a general warm up.

Warm Up Guidelines

The aim of my general warm up is to break a sweat. How long this will take will be influenced by room or environmental conditions, your clothing, and your overall conditioning. I believe somewhere between ten to twenty (10-20) minutes of a large muscle group activity.

I lean towards the stationary bike because it does the job without being too demanding, but am open to any activity based on your needs and situation. It may be a walk - if so, make it longer than the cycle. It may be a jog - in which case you could make it shorter than the cycle duration recommended. Another reason I like the bike is the opportunity to start the knee load easy, without body weight or the impact of gravity, and increase it progressively (provided that the bike you are using allows this). The bike also offers a high number of reps of flexion and extension of the knee, more conducive to bringing out the lubrication in this joint.

So here is what I recommend, breaking the decision into the following three categories of training :

- **Lower body** : Ten to twenty (10-20) minutes of a large muscle group activity e.g. cycling.
- **Upper body trunk** : Optional; if any, five to fifteen (5-15) minutes of a large muscle group activity e.g. cycling.
- **Upper body extremities** : Not needed.

Should you have a desire for more volume in the general warm up, including say to burn more energy, you can increase the duration or frequency of use of this activity.

Note that should you have a desire for more volume in the general warm up, including say to burn more energy, you can increase the duration or frequency of use of this activity. The warm up is a variable for you to manipulate!

Passive Strategies to Enhance and Support the Warm Up

I am going to share with you some really powerful yet simple passive warm up techniques. So simple I don't understand why they are overlooked or ignored by so many. But don't you fall into this trap. Use them!

I will share them in relation to the following :

- o Lower body
- o Upper body.

With all of these recommendations you need to consider your room temperature. If you are in a really hot environment, use the following sparingly. I don't want to see you fry! Use common sense!   There is no advantage to overheating! Rather, there will be a price to pay.

Lower Body

I am an advocate of wearing **sweat suit pants** (or track pants, depending on your vocabulary!) prior to and during the lower body session. This will raise and maintain elevation of the hip and knee joint temperatures. Because of the potential joint wear that these joints experience I feel this is important. Now you can buy different levels of thickness in the material of these pants. In a hotter climate, ensure you have single lined, light material pants that allow some ventilation. In a colder climate you may want or need the double lined material.

I also strongly recommend wearing knee sleeves under or over the track pants.

I also strongly recommend wearing **knee sleeves** under or over the track pants. These are neoprene type material, and are not tight per se. Not so loose either that they slip down. They are fantastic at raising and maintaining an elevated knee temperature, so critical for reducing patella-femoral joint wear (between the knee cap and thigh bone).

The use of knee wraps may replace knee sleeves, but they are more a performance enhancement issue. The knee sleeves are an injury prevention tool.

In between sets, provided the temperature is not too high, I will place a **towel over my shoulders**. This serves two purposes – firstly it maintains body temperature between lifts, and secondly it allows the neural adaptation associated with the flight or fight response when removed.

The longer the rest period between work sets, the more critical it is to maintain body and joint temperature. If you allow your body temperature to lower too much between sets, it affects your arousal level, and your ability to recruit high threshold motor units and fibers. If the temperature of the room is already high, I may delay putting this towel on until the body temperature drops down to what I have established roughly as my minimum, and then put it on. The key is to have it on at least for 30 seconds before the start of the set, so you capture that arousal elevation associated with removing it.

When you remove the towel just before the start of the work set, your body is hit with the room temperature, which will be lower than the temperature you created with the towel around your shoulders. This is like a slap across the face – it gives you body a shock, albeit a small one, but enough to assist you in the elevation of your arousal levels and therefore your ability to perform short, intense work.

When you remove the towel just before the start of the work set, your body is hit with the room temperature. This is like a slap across the face

Both of the above go on before the warm up, and stay on to the end of the workout!

Upper Body

I will always start a workout wearing two or more layers of clothing. The only question for me is how many layers should I start with! And they go on, as above, before the start of the warm up. When they come off is more variable than the lower body options described above.

I always train in a T-shirt, rarely if ever in a singlet. But that is more about the psychology of training than the temperature. Over that t-shirt, I will always commence with a t-shirt material based **long sleeve or 'three-quarter' length**

sleeve. This is a like a t-shirt but the sleeves are long, ending somewhere between the elbow and the wrist.

This will come off as late as possible during the workout. When I say as late as possible, I mean that once my body temperature hits what I call roughly my ceiling of acceptable temperature, it has to come off. What is that temperature? Whatever time you feel that the heat is uncomfortable and negatively impacting on your ability to train.

Now you can also remove it for a set, and replace it during the rest periods. This is an option. You will really feel the temperature change upon removing it, and this can really enhance the arousal levels for the work set.

If the room temperature is cold, I will add **a jumper or sweat suit top** over the three-quarter sleeve t-shirt. This will also come off when I feel that the temperature it is creating is damaging to the workout.

If the room temperature is cold, I will add a jumper or sweat suit top over the three-quarter sleeve t-shirt.

Yes, you could take the sweat suit top off for the work set and return it for the rest periods.

I also strongly recommend the **towel on the shoulders** in the rest periods, as outlined earlier.

There is also neoprene or similar wraps for specific joints, such as the **elbow joint sleeve**, and **shoulder sleeve**. These have a place where you may have chronic injury issues, contributing to raising and maintaining an elevated joint temperature in these joints.

Chapter 8
The Stretch
A performance advantage!

I do two things that are still considered relatively unique. I recommend stretching, and I recommend stretching before the workout. Why is this unique? Because I feel that fear of the unknown is still leaving many advocating avoidance of stretching. You may ask why I say fear of the unknown? I claim that most still don't know what stretching can do! And of those that do support stretching, many have been led to believe that stretching before the workout is 'bad'. At least that is the 'current' thinking. The reasons provided by the anti-stretch advocates change every few years!

I feel that that fear of the unknown is still leaving many advocating avoidance of stretching.

I have been personally stretching in training for nearly four decades now. I have been recommending and enforcing it to large populations of athletes for nearly two decades. I have watched the impact, fine-tuned the application, and found ways to optimize the training results from stretching. I have also learnt the side-effects from not stretching, not stretching enough, or not stretching effectively. In fact, the real world laboratory that I have been fortunate to have participated in has taught me so much about the role of flexibility training!

During this time, I have watched those wishing to influence social behavior generally and specifically in physical training adopt various, transient positions. During the 1980's static stretching (where you hold a stretch for a pre-determined period of time) was considered acceptable, but dynamic stretching (which involves limb or joint movement at varying speeds) was considered unacceptable, even bad! Scientific conclusions regarding static stretching at this time were that 5-30 second stretching holds, repeated 2-3 times, were ideal and adequate.

In the late 1980's and early 1990's I witnessed the rise of a paradigm that suggested you shouldn't stretch too much because if you got too flexible, you would be injury prone i.e. your increased flexibility would result in a higher incidence or chance of being injured.

Then in the mid-1990s, the dominant theme became stretching is acceptable but it can't prevent injuries in the workout so you are wasting your time doing it anyway. In this era dynamic stretching was considered 'good' and static was considered 'bad', a complete turn-around from the decade before. Doesn't the wheel of change occur about every decade?!

By the late 1990s/early 2000's the stretching paradigm was that static stretching had an acute (short-term) impact of reducing your strength, so if you want to do it, only do it afterward the workout. This paradigm suggested more dynamic or PNF (i.e. proprio-neuromuscular facilitation, a special mix of static and dynamic stretching) type stretching should be done before the workout, but again only short duration holds were apparently needed. And as few took stretching seriously enough very few clear and strongly recommend principles existed in mainstream.

During the last few decades so few of the athletic and general training population have taken stretching seriously enough or participated in it enough to have even noticed these paradigm shifts!

So over the last twenty years all I have seen are reasons why you shouldn't stretch! I have witnessed first hand a society, badly in need of improved flexibility, being discouraged from stretching. And when it has been applied, it has for the most part been applied in a manner that was ineffectual and a waste of time. Which reinforces the conclusion that stretching has no real contribution to make and the cycle continues!

This misinformation is not surprising when you see some of the most outspoken people on stretching, who have never personally mastered stretching, never closely assessed the training impact it has had with large sample sizes over many years – yet form dogmatic opinions based on, well, I am not sure what!

I really don't care what type of stretching a person uses, provided they achieve what I believe to be a minimum or optimum range needed to reduce injury potential and enhance performance. Now when I say 'what I believe' I know this is a subjective conclusion, but at least I have formed an opinion - based on my years of empirical observations and personal experiences. It is this I share with you. I am not going to use my time in the dubious pursuit of negating the current themes of 'why you shouldn't stretch' etc. I want to use my time more effectively!

I really don't care what type of stretching a person uses, provided they achieve what I believe to be a minimum or optimum range needed to reduce injury potential and enhance performance.

In this chapter the areas I will address include :

- ❏ Rationale for Stretching
- ❏ Types of Stretching
- ❏ Guidelines for Stretching
- ❏ Keys to Successful Stretching
- ❏ Sample Stretching Program

Rationale for stretching

So why stretch? My rationale for stretching includes :

- o To maintain a specific joint relationships, to keep the joint healthy.
- o To obtain greater joint angles in your strength exercises.
- o To support/accelerate recovery.

To maintain a specific joint relationships

This is my number one reason for stretching. Put simply, if the bones get drawn closer together than desirable, the impingement of connective tissue at the joint can cause all sorts of problems, especially nerve pinching - this can set off all types of neural activity which translates as muscle spasm through to feelings that the muscle has been torn.

You can have a reduction in muscle function due to changes in joint relationships – and you don't necessarily even know it. This can occur before measurable discomfort occurs. And joint surface changes can also commence before you experience or acknowledge the pain. Pain inhibits function.

If the bones get drawn closer together than desirable, the impingement of connective tissue at the joint can cause all sorts of problems, especially nerve pinching.

In addition to the performance enhancement benefits, your joint health is at risk. Two of the most critical joints in strength training are the hip joint (where the femur or upper leg meets the hip bone) and the shoulder (where the humerus or upper arm meets the shoulder joint).

It makes little difference how big and strong you get in the short term, if in the long term you are physically limited because you allowed the joint to become damaged. Joint damage will be accelerated if the joint gap or relationship (distance between two bones) changes.

To obtain greater joint angles in your strength exercises

My second reason for stretching will be to allow you to obtain greater joint angles in your strength exercises that will provide greater training effects e.g. greater hypertrophy, strength at specific joint angles. Anyone wanting to confirm this theory just needs to have say a small muscle like the tibialis anterior (front shin muscle) loosened off and you will see (in most cases) an automatic increase in squat range. If this doesn't work for you, bring in the big guns and stretch the hip flexors extensively. Then squat. You will know what

I am speaking of from experience - which is much more valuable than just reading my opinion about it!

Stretching doesn't need to be performed ahead of training to maintain the joint relationship. This will occur simply as a function or ratio of how much stretching is being done to how much training is being done. However, if you don't have that additional range before the training session, you cannot train the muscle through that range! You miss hypertrophy opportunities. You miss strength adaptations at those new joint angles. And you may be denied the ability to attain desired joint angles for optimal technique.

Even if your pre-training stretching was to make you 'weak' as one of the more dominant recent paradigms suggest (and I am not convinced that this conclusion is accurate), would this negate the benefits to be gained by having the range pre-training? That question is far from being answered.

Unless you have a better idea on how to do it, get into it. And until you give it at least three or so months, how would know anyway?

Bottom line - my stretching methods have been associated with incredibly favorable responses from large numbers of athletes. Unless you have a better idea on how to do it, get into it. And until you give it at least three or so months, how would you know anyway? Would you make your decide on the basis of a particular theory provided by theoreticians?!

To support/accelerate recovery

There is more support for this rationale than the above two. Stretching can really accelerate the recovery process. Not because it 'gets rid of lactic acid'! That's a bit simplistic! Yes, it can improve circulation, and that includes more than blood (e.g. lymph and other fluids). But more importantly I believe it returns a more appropriate length and tension to the muscle.

Now stretching alone is not likely to give you all you need in remodeling of connective tissue and length. I support massage to add to this, and more critically in tissues that are harder to stretch e.g. the ITB (ilio-tibial band, on the outside of the upper leg).

Its contribution to recovery is another reason often provided to support the theory that stretching should be done primarily post-training (e.g. after the workout). True, post-training stretching may be effective in accelerating recovery. But is it much more effective doing it immediately post-training compared to within the following 24 hrs? Is it a reason adequate in itself to negate the benefit of pre-training stretching? I don't believe so. Additionally, I don't believe the body and mind are always in the best state to stretch post-training in a manner that will allow all stretching adaptations and benefits to be obtained. Why? After training, when you are tired and hungry, I question this as an optimal condition for any training!

I don't believe the body and mind are always in the best state to stretch post-training in a manner that will allow all stretching adaptations and benefits to be obtained.

Types of Stretching

Improvements in flexibility may result from any or a combination of the following types of stretching exercises :

- o Static stretching
- o Dynamic stretching
- o PNF (proprio-neuromuscular facilitation) stretching

Static Stretching

Static stretching involves you maintaining a stretch position for certain duration of time. Most textbooks talk 5-60 seconds per rep. I have a different approach. I like to be in the stretch for a lot longer, but rather than come out, generally speaking I will do variations of the stretch within the stretch, which allow me to go further into the stretch. So you may call my stretching techniques a variation on static stretching for the most part.

Static stretching was 'in' during the 1980's but 'out' during the 1990s. Who knows when it will return to favor again and who cares! I find it is the most effective practical way to achieve changes or improvements in flexibility. I say practical because I have no doubt PNF stretching is equally or more effective – but not as practical. Generally speaking I recommend your total stretching program consist predominantly of static stretching.

These stretches can be performed individually or with a partner.

Dynamic Stretching

Dynamic stretching involves movement during the stretch. There are many theories put forward for it's alleged superiority, including specificity. However I don't support most of these and find whilst it has a role, it is not the foundation of my stretching program.

There is a definite place for dynamic stretching in the more specific component of the warm up for a dynamic activity.

There is a definite place for dynamic stretching in the more specific component of the warm up for a dynamic activity. For example, kicking style martial artists will have this type of stretching exercises firmly placed in their warm up protocols.

PNF Stretching

PNF is the abbreviated term for proprio-neuromuscular facilitation type stretches. There are a variety of ways to conduct PNF stretches but basically there is a stretch, followed by a contraction, then a relaxation, then a furthering of the stretch position.

This style of stretching probably has the most science support as the most effective way to stretch for improvement in length. It has also gained support recently from the 'stretching before training makes you weak' school of thought.

The reality is that PNF stretching is not always the most practical or time efficient way to stretch. It has a solid place in the program, but in most real-world situations, will not dominate my programs.

These stretches can be performed individually or with a partner.

Guidelines for Stretching

The following variables will be discussed :

The reality is that PNF stretching is not always the most practical or time efficient way to stretch.

- o Duration of the stretching workout
- o Duration of each stretching exercise
- o Order of stretches
- o The tight side rule
- o Progression in stretching

Duration of the Stretching Workout

The most important issue in flexibility training may be total duration i.e. how much time do you spend in the stretch. See the below table for suggestions as to frequency, duration, number of repeats etc.

I make the following generalized recommendations as to the duration of stretching prior to strength training sessions :

- Pre-upper body stretching : 15-20 minutes.
- Pre-lower body stretching : 20-40 minutes.

As for dedicated stretching sessions aimed at accelerating recovery, allowing mediation, or improving flexibility, I usually recommend 60-90 minutes. These sessions, for those serious about their training, should be done 1-2 times a week.

Table 15 – Variables of stretching based on specific needs.

VARIABLES	TYPES OF STRETCHING		
	REHAB-ILITATION (Light)	TRAINING/ COMPETITION PREPARAT-ION (Medium)	INJURY PREVENT (Heavy)
Frequency	Daily	Prior to training or competition	1-3/wk (influenced by training load)
Total Duration	5-10 mins	10-30 mins	30-90 mins (influenced by training load)
Repeats (per exercise)	1-5	2-4	3-6
Duration of Repeats	30 sec - 5 mins	10-30 secs	30 sec - 10 mins
Number of Exercises	1-4	6-12	8-20
Comments	insert in daily routine to avoid missing	do prior to or following training	select a comfortable location with no distractions, relax

For dedicated stretching sessions aimed to at accelerating recovery, allowing mediation, or improving flexibility, I usually recommend 60-90 minutes.

Duration of Each Stretching Exercise

I recommend initially you hold each position for a shorter time than I expect you to be holding them as you get more advanced. The duration of the hold is simply a training variable, part of the progressive overload opportunity. As you adapt, to gain further improvements you need to increase the duration of the stretch. Till how long? I can't say for sure, but I can say this – stretching is the only form of training that I generally believe more is better!

Now this doesn't mean you cannot over-train stretching. You can. Stretching training needs to have the same recovery considerations given to it as any form of training. But unlike many other forms of training, you may benefit from doing more provided you are conditioned to it!

If you plan to stretch for say 30 minutes before lower body strength training, and you had six muscle groups, a literal division may be to say do 5 minutes on each muscle group. Now this is simply a generalization, as some muscle groups will require more time than others, based on their size (the bigger they are the more stretching they may require) or your needs (some may be lagging behind more-so).

This doesn't mean you cannot over-train stretching. You can. Stretching training needs to have the same recovery considerations given to it as any form of training.

Further to that, within a muscle group you may have a few variations of stretches you want to implement. This is how I work out how long I can afford to spend in each stretching exercise or muscle group.

Order of Stretches

There is a rationale to the order I have recommended doing the stretches in. The order basically aims to reduce the limiting factor of the next subsequent stretch. For example, a tight neck (upper trap) can cause impingement symptoms through the shoulder joint, so loosing off the neck first will allow the muscles of the shoulder to 'let go'.

Focus on what you are doing, feeling for the stretch, relaxing into them. You can reverse this lowering of arousal in your warm up sets, so don't panic about this.

The Tight Side Rule

Most people will have one side that is tighter than the other side e.g. left hamstring tighter than the right hamstring. I have developed a method of addressing this imbalance, based on an acute understanding of the power of sequence. Basically, the side you stretch first gets longer and better focus than the side you stretch second!

So once you work out which is your tighter side in each muscle group, do the tighter side first. Then consider repeating the tighter side again e.g. order would go tighter side, looser side, and tighter side.

Progression in Stretching

Stretching should be conducted as per your strength training – monitoring progress from session to session, aiming to increase range from session to session. Too often stretching is seen as something to be done without applying the base training principles such as progressive overload.

Most people will have one side that is tighter than the other side e.g. left hamstring tighter than the right hamstring. I have developed a method of addressing this imbalance.

This is in part because few know how to treat stretching with the respect it deserves. Flexibility, along with speed, strength and endurance, is one of the four dominant physical qualities. It can and should be treated with the same respect as the other three, and by using the same training principles as any form of training.

So don't just go through the motions! Note your range – aim to improve it from session to session. Use it to gauge your recovery and readiness to train. If a given muscle group is too tight, spend more time on it until it is to the level that is safe and effective to train. In some cases, you may even cancel whole of part of your session based on the information you gathered during the stretch. There is so much power in the stretching session!

Keys to Successful Stretching

To achieve the best result in flexibility training it is more than simply putting in the hours. Using some of the "Keys to Stretching" listed below may enhance your training results.

- **Warm up first** : Look to break a sweat prior to stretching - it will increase the pliability of the connective tissue. That doesn't mean you cannot stretch cold. It just means that if you stretch after raising your body temperature, you will start with greater range.

- **Focus** : Stretching to improve length of connective tissue should be treated the same as any other type of training where improvement is the goal. Would you hold an irrelevant conversation with a friend whilst performing skill training with a specialist coach? Give stretching your complete attention during these stretching sessions. Also select a venue where you will minimize the distractions.

Relaxing is a critical component in static stretching where the goal is to improve the length of the connective tissue. If you go too far into the earlier repeats, you will not be able to relax.

- **Relax** : Relaxing is a critical component in static stretching where the goal is to improve the length of the connective tissue. If you go too far into the earlier repeats, you will not be able to relax. As a rule, do not attempt to progress to the next level of range until you have achieved a relaxed state in the position you are in.

- **Breathing** : You can control your breathing to facilitate relaxing. During the exhalation or breathing out phase, focus on relaxing the body.

- **Work at your level** : Don't try to achieve the same apparent range as another person; work at a level appropriate for yourself and look to improve on it.

- **Progress in level of intensity with each repeat** : When performing the first repeat of any stretch, work within a comfortable range; in the second repeat, look to move further; and again in the third repeat, look to go further. If doing three repeats, only the third repeat should be challenging i.e. a mild to moderate degree of discomfort. If doing five repeats, the fourth and fifth repeat may would be likewise.

- **Avoid inappropriate pain** : It is important to recognize that not all the stretching exercises will suit everyone, and that even with one individual, circumstances change. A simple guideline that can be stressed is that if it causes inappropriate discomfort, look for an alternative. Learn to recognize between a mild to moderate stretching sensation and higher level of pain, and avoid the latter.

- **Do not compromise the correct technique**: Whilst every different position has a specific stretch response, many of the stretching exercises are taught initially in the most effective position from a general standpoint. e.g. the position of the hips in the hamstring and quadriceps exercises. Remember it is the degree of stretch obtained that is important, not how far you appear to have stretched.

If you identify that one side of your body is tighter that the other, perform this side first. This ensures that the tight side is prioritized.

- **Tighter side first** : If you identify that one side of your body is tighter that the other, perform this side first. This ensures that the tight side is prioritized.

- **Ballistic stretching after static stretching** : Static stretching is very effective in improving the length of the connective tissue. However there is a place for ballistic or dynamic stretching, especially in sports where the limbs are involved in high speed movements at end of range. Ballistic stretching may be required prior to training or competition, and may best be performed after some static stretching.

- **Good communication between partners in paired stretching** : Especially when PNF techniques are used.

Sample Stretching Program

The following are sample static stretching programs that you can use both pre and post training, and in any additional stretching workout during the week. Note that you only need to stretch the muscles and joints you will be using in that workout e.g. bench press day – no need to do lower body.

However, be mindful that when going heavy, you may benefit from stretching ALL muscles and joints involved. For example, when using an arch in the bench press, I do prepare the lower back by stretching. When going heavy in the squat I do prepare the shoulder joint, especially the chest. When doing snatches, I would always prepare the shoulder joint.

If you have arthritic shoulders you will want to start the arm circles slowly and in smaller circles, progressing to a faster movement and bigger circles.

The following sample static stretching programs include :

- o Sample Stretches for Before an Upper Body Workout
- o Sample Stretches for Before a Lower Body Workout

Sample Stretches for Before an Upper Body Workout

- **Arm swings** : One hand at a time, swing the arm in circles from front to back 10 times, then back to front 10 times to the side of the body. Do the same on the other side. If you have arthritic shoulders you will want to start the arm circles slowly and in smaller circles, progressing to a faster movement and bigger circles. There is also an arm swing motion across the front of the body that I use as a pre-activity for the above as it is even less stressful on the joint.

- **Neck stretches** : Place one hand by the body. Lower the head the other way, and use the hand of the side that the head is leaning towards to pull the head gently over further, taking the ear to the shoulder. Then do the same in reverse on the other side. Repeat the tightest side. There is another option for those keen to enhance this area, and that is to take the ear towards the chest, stretching the broader upper trap area to across closer to the spine.

- **Shoulder stretch** : This is an old standby - there are three positions : i. arm up over the head, other hand pulling backwards on the triceps just above the elbow, stretching the triceps; ii. arm across the front of the chest, other arm pulling it in to the body from that same leverage point on the tricep just above the elbow, stretching the posterior or rear of the shoulder and compressing the acromio-clavicular joint; iii. arm up behind the body, other hand also behind the body pulling it up, stretching the anterior or front of the shoulder.

- **Forearm stretches** : Place one arm straight in front of the body. Use the other hand to assist in creating the stretch. There are 3 positions I recommend - i. palm up, pull the hand down, stretching the forearm flexors; ii. palm down, pull the hand up, stretching the forearm extensors; iii. (read this carefully now!) the palm of one hand faces down, then rotates outwards, and then upwards - the palm of the other hand then contacts with the back of this hand, pulling the fingers further around and up, stretching the forearm rotators.

Note that you only need to stretch the muscles and joints you will be using in that workout e.g. bench press day – no need to do lower body.

- **Chest stretch** : Stand close to a vertical frame or door frame, and have one hand up on this frame. There are 4 positions: i. elbow bent to 90 degrees, upper arm parallel to the ground, lower arm in contact with vertical frame, rotate the body away - this should provide a very isolated chest stretch; ii. now move a bit further away from the frame and extend the arm until the elbow is just bent, hand and/or wrist in contact with frame, palm facing forward, rotate body away - this will still be a strong chest stretch, but now will also be felt in the biceps; iii. now move a litter further from the wall again and straighten the arm out completely, hand/wrist still in contact with palm facing forward, rotate away - this will increase the stretch in the biceps/forearm; iv. keeping the arm straight, rotate the forearm taking the palm down and then facing to the rear, rotate away - this will take the stretch also into the forearm extensors.

- **Lat stretch** : There are two here; i. stand under a horizontal frame such as a chin bar, but make sure your feet can still touch the ground; hold the bar above you with one arm at a time, lowering your body down and pushing the pelvis in the opposite direction to get a stretch on the lats; ii. stand in front of a vertical frame and lean forward, grasping it with one hand; the upper body is basically parallel to the ground now; rotate the hips away from the stretch side, to get a stretch down the lats and upper back.

Static stretching is very effective in improving the length of the connective tissue.

Sample Stretches for Before a Lower Body Workout

- **Calf stretch** : There are two positions for this - i. stand in front of a wall or vertical frame, placing one foot at about a 45 degree angle up the wall, with the heel still in contact with the ground; keeping the leg straight, look to move the hips towards the wall; ii. keeping the same position, bent the stretch-side leg at the knee; you may want to kneel the other knee onto the ground; now focus on moving the knee towards the wall or vertical frame. This second position will shift the stretch lower towards the heel.

- **Lower back** : Lie on your back on the ground; there are a few positions for this stretch, but only go beyond the first position if your back has had no recent trauma; i. bring your knees to your chest, pulling them into the chest by levering your arms under the knee joint; rock gently; ii. now extend the legs until they are straight and then slowly take the legs over the head as far as you can comfortably go (if you feel this more in the upper back or neck, be sensible about how far you take this position); iii. now bend the knees, looking to take the knees towards the ground either side of the ears. Whichever position you go to, be careful and remember to go slow when coming out of the position.

- **Hamstrings** : Still on your back, there are a few positions you can use - i. use your towel as a stirrup under one foot, keeping this leg straight, take the leg up as high as the hamstring will allow it; ii. drop the towel out, bend this leg, and use your hands to pull around the ankles, bringing the slightly bent knee as close to the chest as you can; iii. place the opposite side arm under the knee joint, pulling the knee as close to the body as you can, and the same side hand pulling from behind the heel, bringing the foot as close to the shoulders as you can.

- **Gluteal** : Still on your back, there are a few positions you can use - i. lift one leg, bent at the knee and take the lower leg across the body; with the same-side hand, push the knee away, and with the opposite hand pull the foot towards the head; ii. take the foot across to the other hip, holding the ankle with the opposite side hand. With the same side hand, pull the knee across your body towards the opposite shoulder; iii. now lift the non-stretching leg up until the stretching leg is pressed up against the bottom of the quads; take the same side hand through the 'd shape' formed by both legs ('through the hole') and the opposite side hand goes down and pulls the non-stretch side leg up towards the chest by holding onto the top of the shin, just below the knee.

- **Posterior chain** : Still on your back, there are two positions - i. lift one leg up straight in the air, then lower it down over the other side of the body, keeping the leg straight; your degree of flexibility will determine what angle relative to the body it goes

There is a place for ballistic or dynamic stretching, especially in sports where the limbs are involved in high speed movements at end of range.

down; progressively lift the leg up towards the head, keeping the leg straight; ii. now bend the stretch side leg, pulling the bent knee down to the ground using the opposite side hand.

Note that you only need to stretch the muscles and joints you will be using in that workout.

- **Hip flexor/quads** : Kneel on the ground in front of and facing away from a low bench, with one foot on the ground in front of you and the other foot up on the bench behind you. The foot up on the bench behind you has the knee on that same leg resting on the ground. Place your towel rolled up under the knee as a cushion. The stretch side leg has the knee bent, knee on the towel, and foot up on the bench behind you. There are two positions I recommend you work through : i. the first position requires you to take your gluts (butt!) towards the stretch side heel. If this is easy, add the 'pelvic tilt' i.e. suck the top of the pelvis in or backwards, and push the bottom end of the pelvis forward; ii. now take the foot of the non-stretch leg out further away from the bench, keep the chest up (try putting your hands on your head) and lower your pelvis down as low as it can go (your stretch side foot is still up on the bench behind).

Recommended Reference Material

Ian King's Guide To Individual Stretching – available at www.getbuffed.net
Flexibility Training Video Series   - available at www.kingsports.net
Flexibility Specialization Video Series - available at www.kingsports.net

Chapter 9
The Abdominal Exercises

Neglect these at your peril!

Most people agree that abdominal training is important. That is however about where the consensus ends. What specific exercises, what loading parameters, when should they be done – these are all variables or questions subject to greater variety in beliefs. For me the most important aspect is not what anyone believes should be done – rather, what is being achieved. Are their abdominals adequately strong or functioning? From my observations, the answer is no. I see a lot of paper tigers – people with incredible amounts of knowledge and even strong beliefs - but little positive results!

The most important aspect is not what anyone believes should be done – rather, what is being achieved.

I believe that I can provide you with something that whilst may not give you any consensus with your friends opinions, will give you results worth training for! In sharing this with you, I will address :

- ❑ Rationale for Abdominal Training
- ❑ Historical Trends in Abdominal Training
- ❑ Abdominal Sub-Categories
- ❑ Guidelines for Abdominal Training
- ❑ Notes Regarding the Abdominal Training Program in *Get Buffed!* ™ II (Get More Buffed!)

Rationale for Abdominal Training

There are a number of reasons why you may be or should be doing abdominal exercises and they include:

- o Abdominal training and visual impact
- o Abdominal training and transfer to sport
- o Abdominal training and injury prevention

Abdominal training and visual impact : The majority of people training with strength training would be pursuing this specific goal in relation to their abdominal training. But whether the high volumes of abdominal training being performed by some will give them the desired appearance is not as clear. If for no other reason the fact that the subcutaneous fat in the abdominal region will block the appearance. Will the abdominal training selectively reduce this body fat? Most say no, I say maybe not but I am open to theories on this. I am not convinced the jury's verdict is fully complete in this area.

Whether application of sports specific abdominal training has superiority over non-specific abdominal training combined with on-field specific training is also unclear.

What I can say with greater conviction is that there is potential for improved visual impact if the abdominal are kept in a shortened state through strength training.

Abdominal training and transfer to sport : The contribution of abdominal training to sport has received no shortage of press but I suggest that many principles are misguided. For one, the statement that *'a strong mid-section is needed to transfer the force from the lower body to the upper body'* is nice but perhaps unsubstantiated. Secondly, whether application of sports specific abdominal training has superiority over non-specific abdominal training combined with on-field specific training is also unclear. Additionally, appropriate periodization from low level of difficulty to higher level of difficulty is often overlooked in the pursuit of immediate application of apparently specific exercises.

Basically I feel that the performance enhancement aspects of abdominal training are over-rated and the injury prevention aspects are under-rated. Sure lip service is given to injury prevention through abdominal training, but I question the value of most exercises given for this purpose. And in the area of performance enhancement, I question the transfer. Especially from the so-called 'more specific' exercises.

For example, not too many sports are conducted on plastic, air filled surfaces....We are in an era of finding the holy grail of specificity, and the performance of the sporting activity is neglected. The strength and conditioning profession are as much to blame as anyone (and of all professionals should know better) for promoting this over-reliance on off-field exercise to achieve on-court success. Anything that is off the court/field/sporting arena is what I call non-specific anyway!

I don't use strength training to gain specificity. For me, it is the physical quality (speed, strength, endurance and flexibility) that generally speaking can and should be performed with the lowest degree of relative specificity and which result in the greatest transfer. Don't aim to sell me on the specificity of an off-court activity – I just want to know the transfer!

The role of the abdominal and other trunk stabilizers has received appropriate attention in therapy and injury prevention studies.

Abdominal training and injury prevention : Abdominal training for injury prevention is not a new concept. For example, strength writer of an earlier era, Charles Mac Mahon, was writing about the value of strong abdominals and other trunk stabilizers for injury prevention - in 1931! (Everyone has a weak spot physically, *Correct Eating – Strength, Vol. XVI(6)*, p. 38-40). The role of the abdominal and other trunk stabilizers has received appropriate attention in therapy and injury prevention studies. This information has yet to fully filter down however, based on the incidence of injuries that can be attributed to inappropriately prepared abdominal and trunk stabilizer muscles.

I feel that the primary purpose of abdominal training is to contribute to the health of the lower back, hips and lower extremities. Therefore most abdominal training I provide, including this program, is prioritized towards injury prevention.

Historical Trends in Abdominal Training

The historical emphasis may have been biased towards the performance of trunk flexion, which we will call dominantly an 'upper abdominal' exercise. Take for example a general strength circuit used by the US Marine Corps Physical Fitness Academy, Quantico, Virginia, in the 1960s (Rasch, P.J. 1966, *Weight Training*, Wm C Brown Co Publishers, Iowa). In a one exercise per major muscle group circuit, straight leg, anchored sit-ups were chosen.

The historical emphasis may have been biased towards the performance of trunk flexion.

This is not to suggest that there has been a lack of awareness of the multi-functional and multi-directional role of the abdominals. Bill Starr in his 1976 classic 'The Strongest Shall Survive' wrote that the abdominals '...can be strengthened in a wide variety of ways. Sit-ups of all types, leg raises, trunk rotation movements all involve the abdominal muscles to different degree..." Bill Pearls 1986 classic "Keys to the Inner Universe" list and graphically illustrates over 100 exercises.

The knowledge and the practice seem to be gapped. I still see exercise programs that select only one abdominal exercise, usually a trunk flexion movement.

In many circles, including para or quasi-medical (disciplines/occupations aligned with or attempting to align with the medical profession), there has been a trend towards conservative prescription in abdominal training, led by the paradigm that any involvement of the hip flexors in hip or trunk flexion is bad, and there only limited range trunk flexion is acceptable.

When sport scientists first analyzed the 'unanchored' straight leg setup many decades ago, the conclusion was that the iliopsoas and other hip flexors were too involved. The concern here was inadequate stimulation of the other abdominal muscles and the injury potential of the anterior shear on the lumbar vertebrae. Since those observations there has been an out of control drive to find and exclusively use exercises with no hip flexor involvement. Hip flexor involvement isn't bad!

There is definitely an argument for strengthening the abdominals in isolation. The periodization of the abdominal training should consider a progression from isolation towards integration. Lack of exposure to compound movements (involving more than one joint and muscle) can create a functional weakness in itself. The aerobic industry was one sector responsible for advancing the myth of isolation only abdominal exercises.

Hip flexor involvement isn't bad!

I believe this politically correct movement has gone to far, and provided they can be performed safely in any given individual, generally recommend full range sit-ups in trunk flexion.

A more recent trend to emerge is the Swiss ball trend, where the dominant paradigm is that only those abdominal exercises performed on this training tool are effective. The Swiss ball, in my mind, has been over-rated. This is not to suggest that it isn't a nice toy, but generally speaking it has been over-promoted.

Here's some of the dogma I have seen over the last 10-20 years :

- Never do straight leg sit-ups.
- Hip flexor involvement is bad so only crunch up a few degrees.
- Weak abs prevent transfer of force from lower to upper body.

- Doing abs on your back is a waste of time as it is not specific.
- Swiss ball abdominal training is more specific.
- Lower abdominals are always weaker than upper. ·
- You cannot separate lower and upper abdominals in training.
- Only do high rep abdominal training.
- Only do low rep abdominal training.
- Never do abdominal training at the start of the workout.

Personally, I don't buy into any of the above. There is a time and a place for everything. The reality is, most of what each of us perceive as our reality is based on our previous personal experiences or observations. My conclusions are also based on my experiments with athletes more than experiments on my own. I like the bigger sample size. But don't go thinking that because I write a sample program one way means that's the only way I do it! Rest assured I take all the variables and play with them differently in different situations.

There is a time and a place for everything.

Abdominal Sub-Categories

I divide the abdominal muscle groups or functions down into six (6). The technical correctness of my divisions I will leave to those with the time and motivation to debate to do so. This is a simple and effective approach to ensuring exposure to all abdominal and some of the other trunk stabilizers :

o Hip Flexion
o Trunk Flexion
o Rotation
o Lateral Flexion
o Co-contraction of Abs and Gluts
o Integrated

Hip Flexion

Hip flexion involves the hips moving towards the trunk. There is empirical evidence to suggest the belief of most in the therapy/rehab field that majority of people have weaker hip flexors than trunk flexors, due to the bias in the history of abdominal training towards trunk flexion.

Perhaps the most popular **hip flexion** ('lower abdominal') exercise is the knee up drill, done either with a low pulley or on an incline or at extreme, vertically (i.e. hanging from a chin bar or similar). I see little value in doing any abdominal exercise that exceeds your ability to selectively recruit the desired muscle groups in the desired joint positions. Hip flexion drills deserve this conservative 'selective recruitment' approach the most of all the six categories I define because of the direct potential involvement of the hip flexors. Stresses on the lower back are greatest in these drills of all abdominal drills.

The 'thin tummy drill' is the corner stone I build my abdominal programs upon.

My preference is to master a drill I call **'thin tummy'**. This is not an easy drill to teach. I have a preference for teaching it on your back, knees bent to 90 degrees, feet flat. You may however see it also taught in a kneeling position.

Lie on your back and place your little finger on your stomach in the groove between your thigh and trunk, underneath the belt line. Have your thumbs on your upper tummy. First, 'suck' your tummy inwards, making your abdominal circumference as thin as you can (just imagine you are on the beach!) and then attempt to recruit the abdominal muscles under your little fingers i.e. the 'lower abdominals'. Minimize or avoid upper abdominal contraction and definitely no bulging of the upper tummy. You must maintain that 'thin dish'. Initially you may struggle to even find the muscles I want you to contract! Work with 5-second holds, 10 reps a set, and the next step is to be able to breath normally during the isometric contractions!

The 'thin tummy drill' is the corner stone I build my abdominal programs upon, so yes, I believe it should be mastered first and foremost.

Trunk Flexion

Trunk flexion involves the trunk moving towards the hips. Even though there is empirical evidence to confirm the bias in the history of abdominal training towards trunk flexion has left this abdominal sub-category stronger than other abdominal sub-categories, most people I see are grossly inefficient in this area.

I am not going to please the 'hyper-functionalists' because the above two examples were on your back on the ground, and so are the next few!

Perhaps the most popular abdominal drill for the 'upper abdominal' or **trunk flexion** is a variation of the setup e.g. weight plate on chest sit-ups. My base exercise for this abdominal category is what I call the **'slow up/slow down'**. Lie on the ground with your knees bent to 90 degrees, feet flat, hands parallel to the ground by your side. Then sit up slowly, taking 5 seconds to sit up fully. This phase should be performed using a constant speed (i.e. no acceleration) and in the absence of momentum from other body parts (which is one of the reasons I ask the arms to remain straight and parallel to the grounds during the setup). Then take 5 seconds to lower back down, again with no change in speed of movement. If you are unable to perform a full range setup in this manner i.e. at this speed, with no additional momentum, and feet staying down – there are lower levels, with less demanding options.

I am not going to please the 'hyper-functionalists' because the above two examples were on your back on the ground, and so are the next few!

Rotation

Rotation can involve trunk or hip rotation or both. They involve the hip or trunk rotating along the long axis of the body. Note this rotation can involve either the trunk (which is more common) or the legs.

This movement is not seen as often as the above two sub-categories. When it is performed, at least traditionally in strength training, it is often performed in a manner with limited external resistance. This raises questions about the benefits of the movement. The movement that I refer to is the traditional movement in bodybuilding where you sit on a bench with a broomstick or back on the shoulders and rotate.

Arguably the **Russian Twist** is the most popular trunk rotation drill. Sit on the ground with knees bent to 90 degrees and lean your trunk back to 45 degrees. Keeping this trunk angle, and with arms out straight, fingers interlocked, and arms maintained at 90 degrees to the upper body, rotate the trunk from the waist (not the shoulders!). To increase the level of difficulty I like to use a concurrent alternate leg cycle (so that the legs never touch the ground). Of course you can add an external load (weight plate or medicine ball) to the hands, but I don't feel this is necessary for most when the drill is performed in a controlled fashion (e.g.. 202), and later down the sequence of abdominal drills.

Arguably the Russian Twist is the most popular trunk rotation drill.

Remember, rotation drills for the lower body can be performed in addition to or instead of upper body rotational drills.

Lateral Flexion

These drills involve the trunk flexing along the frontal plane. For example, the shoulders being brought closer to the hips, maintaining the front on plane of the body.

Lateral flexion drills are less commonly witnessed in the gym but the most popular ones you will see include the side raise off the end of the Roman Chair or a bench, or standing low pulley or single DB lateral trunk bends. I think the lateral trunk flexion off the end of a bench is the king of these exercises, especially when you add a twist. But for starters, I like to use the simple, controlled drill of 'side raises on the ground'.

Lie on your back, bending both knees to 90 degrees. Then, keeping the knees together, roll them to one side so that the outside of the lower knee is in contact with the ground. Touch the forehead with the fingers of each arm, and have the elbows motionless at 45 degrees from the head. Take 2-3 seconds to flex or sit up as far as you can (which wont be far!). Pause for a second at the top, then lower down in 2-3 seconds. Do 10-30 reps on one side, before repeating the same on the other side. This is nowhere near as demanding as the side raises off the end of a bench, but if you sequence this drill low in the abdomen workout, and use a strict technique, it will do the job!

The co-contraction of the abdominals and gluteals is a drills with greater application to those interested in performance and injury prevention.

Co-contraction of the Abs and Gluts

The co-contraction of the abdominals and gluteals involve focusing on a simultaneous contraction of these two muscles groups. The significance of this is these two muscle groups are responsible for maintaining hip position. This ability is critical in many aspect of lifting and sport, as well as in daily life.

The co-contraction of the abdominals and gluteals is a drills with greater application to those interested in performance and injury prevention. There is no traditional movement of this kind that I am aware off. So to perform my base movement in this category, which I call the 'seated cheek-abdominal squeezes', sit on a bench with your chest up, knees together. Then contract the lower abdominals and gluteals, attempting to 'levitate' up from the bench as high as you can. Hold this for 5 seconds, repeated 5-15 times. The next challenge will be to breathe normally during the isometric contraction! You can have your fingers placed on the lower / outer abdominals during this to act as a bio-feedback device. This is not a drill that will create a lot of pain or discomfort as you do it, but the value is significant yet subtle.

Integrated

Integrated abdominal drills involve using multiple abdominal sub-categories as well as many other muscles of the body at the same time.

Many of the exercises used in the above sub-categories use more than one group of muscles. It is the specific goal of this category to involve them all. Many of the drills on the Swiss ball fall within this category. I will however give you a simple drill, requiring no equipment. Go into a push up position on the ground. Keeping the body totally flat (parallel to the ground), and raise one arm up. Ideally raise it to parallel from the ground in front of you, taking 5 seconds from take off to landing. Do the same with other side arm, and then do 5-second holds with one leg up then the other. Now do opposite arm and leg at the same time. You will have performed a total of six five-second reps (6 x 5 seconds). You may wish to repeat this cycle one or more times. Remember to keep the body flat, not allowing the hips to sag down. If a push up position is more than you can handle, work off the knees.

Many of the exercises used in the above sub-categories use more than one group of muscles.

Guidelines for Abdominal Training

In this section I will address :

- o Frequency of Abdominal Training
- o Volume of Abdominal Training
- o Intensity of Abdominal Training
- o Sequence of Abdominal Training Within the Workout
- o Sequencing of the Abdominal Sub-groups
- o Periodization of Abdominal Training

o Abdominal Muscle sub-group Allocation to Training Days
o Integration of Abdominal Training with Other Muscle Groups
o Common Faults in Program Design

Frequency of Abdominal Training

Rather than getting caught up in a discussion as to whether abdominal muscles are phasic (power producing) or tonic (stabilizing contributing), I am going to simply stress the inverse relationship between volume and intensity. Abdominal muscles need to recover also! If your primary concern is injury prevention, I lean towards more frequent lower load (i.e. volume and intensity) exposures. For example, a total of 2-4 sets daily or at least 5 out of 7 days. If your primary concern is to specific power production (e.g.. performance specific), a higher load less frequent exposure may be more effective e.g. 6-10 sets per session, 2-3 days a week. If your focus is injury prevention and visual contribution, a medium load and frequency may be effective e.g.. 3-4 days a week, 3-6 sets per session. (see Table 16)

If your primary concern is injury prevention, I lean towards more frequent lower load (i.e. volume and intensity) exposures.

Volume of Abdominal Training

How many sets of abdominal training should I do? In his 1931 article in *Correct Eating – Strength*, Charles MacMahon wrote : *"...it is surprising, I might add, how little exercise is required to keep the muscles strong enough to prevent (injuries)..."*.

And I have found this also. If injury prevention is your goal, 1-4 sets per workout may be sufficient. If your primary concern is specific power production (e.g. performance specific), a higher volume may be more effective e.g.. 6-10 sets per session. If your focus is injury prevention and visual contribution, an intermediate volume may be more effective e.g. 3-6 sets per session (see Table 17).

Table 16 – Abdominal training goal and recommendations for frequency and load.

Training Goal	Frequency	Load	Example
Injury prevention	5-6/wk days	low	1- 4 sets
Performance Specific	2-3/wk days	high	6-10sets
General	3-4/wk days	med	3- 6 sets
(i.e. visual, injury prevention, performance)			

Intensity of Abdominal Training

We can treat the abdominal muscles much like any other muscles. Going closer to muscle fatigue and failure will increase the fatigue curve, and only do this if you don't plan on training that abdominal muscle group for another 2-3 days. With regard to loading, the lower reps may have a greater training effect on the fast twitch muscle/motor units and the higher reps on the slow twitch muscle/motor units. I match the loading to the specific training goal.

Going closer to muscle fatigue and failure will increase the fatigue curve, and only do this if you don't plan on training that abdominal muscle group for another 2-3 days.

Table 17 – Generalization for load relative to specific training goals in abdominal exercises.

Specific Training Goal	Reps	TUT (sec)
Control/stability	10-30	40-100
General strength	10-20	40-70
Maximal strength	5-15	10-40
Explosive power	5-15	10-40
Strength endurance	20-100	40-100

Sequence of Abdominal Training Within the Workout

The continuing dominant paradigm is that abdominals should be done last. What if they are the weakest body part? That doesn't seem to matter! What if they are the number one training focus for performance? Again it doesn't seem to matter – they are placed last. Why? The repetitive answer I get to this is *'because they cause fatigue of stabilizers and it would be dangerous to do things like squats after doing abdominals'*. Where is the evidence? Is this evidence from empirical observations or 'scientific' research? Again, that doesn't seem to matter. NOBODY does abdominals first! What a load of trash! The excuses support the paradigm, nothing more. I train abdominal first when they are the priority for whatever reason, and only put them to the end of the workout when I don't want to totally avoid any possibility of total body fatigue prior to a maximal strength workout. That is, I wouldn't want the total body fatigue draining the neuro-muscular system, reducing the potential for load. But nothing to do with injury potential!

The continuing dominant paradigm is that abdominals should be done last.

Sequencing of the Abdominal Sub-groups

I apply the priority sequence rule i.e. I find out the weakest to strongest generally speaking, and do them in that order. This is why most programs might show the lower abdominal receiving a higher sequencing in the training week than the lower abdominal – many people have stronger upper abdominal function from a training history biased towards this movement.

Periodization of Abdominal Training

Generally speaking I like to commence a training career, year or block, with the mastering of the 'control' strength sub-quality, and then over time, phase along the sub-quality continuum to my end goal. This is simply moving from left to right along the strength sub-qualities continuum (refer to the

Table below). However if the sub-quality I want to peak with is a sub-quality from earlier along the continuum (back to the left), I return to it for my 'peaking' program.

Table 18 – The strength sub-qualities continuum.

Control/ stability	→	General strength/ hypertrophy	→	Maximal strength	→	Speed strength	→	Strength endurance

Abdominal Muscle Sub-group Allocation to Training Days

If you are training with a day or more rest between sessions, you can afford to do all six (6) sub-groups within the training session. You don't have to, but you can. If you are training two or more days in a row with no day off, then I recommend you do not train all six in the one session. I might allocate abdominal muscle sub-groups in the following way in a 4 day split :

If you are training with a day or more rest between sessions, you can afford to do all six (6) sub-groups within the training session.

Table 19 – Sample abdominal allocation over a week.

A	B	C	D
Lower abdom	Upper abdom	Lower abdom	Upper abdom
Lateral flexion	Rotation	Lateral flexion	Rotation
Co-contraction	Integration	Co-contraction	Integration

Integration of Abdominal Training with Other Muscle Groups

There are very few times when I caution against the mixing of any combination of muscle groups. However there is one combination in relation to the abdominals and this is it - I have found that it is sometimes not wise to place the lower abdominal exercises on lower body days. This is because I feel that many 'lower abdominal' drills have the affect of pulling the top of the pelvis forward (anterior rotation). I don't believe this is an ideal temporary state to be in for the execution of loaded lower extremity exercises such as squats and deadlifts. I prefer therefore to do 'upper abdominal' drills on lower body days.

Common Faults in Program Design

The most common faults I see in abdominal program design include :

I have found that it sometimes not wise to place the lower abdominal exercises on lower body days.

- No abdominal training at all!
- No assessment of weakness/strength or attempts to determine the sequence by priority of need.
- Focus in sequencing and volume on strength, not weakness.
- Use of inappropriately high level of difficulty exercise e.g. getting someone with zero lower abdominal 'control' to perform straight leg raises hanging from a chin-up bar or similar apparatus for this exercise!

Notes Regarding the Abdominal Training Program in *Get Buffed!*™ II (Get More Buffed!)

I know that some of you will want more information about the rationale of the abdominal program in *Get Buffed!*™ II (Get More Buffed!) so here it is – generally speaking this program prioritizes the potential benefits of abdominal training in the following order:

1. Injury prevention
2. Transfer to sport
3. Visual impact

I feel that the primary purpose of abdominal training is to contribute to the health of the lower back, hips and lower extremities. I placed sport transfer second because of the general transfer this program may have. There is no attempt to be sport specific or hyper-specific in the program. For some 'experts' this would negate any potential in this program, but by now you may have learned a few things about my approach – such as I don't go down the hyper-specific path and I don't really care what others think. I review it, take some, and leave the rest. The negative social implications of holding a different opinion became superfluous to me many years ago. The reason I placed visual last is because of the impact of body fat on the visuals of the abdominals. I know of at least one highly promoted abdominal 'wash-board', where they omit to share with the audience the role of liposuction in that particular case!

I have not addressed the posterior trunk muscles, as they are addressed adequately through the other exercises selected in this program.

I feel that the primary purpose of abdominal training is to contribute to the health of the lower back, hips and lower extremities.

I will now expand on the following anticipated questions :

Can I change the order of the exercises? Sure – provided you have an objective rationale for doing do. I have based the programs on the loose assumptions including that most peoples 'lower abdominals' will be less advanced than their upper abdominals. This is not always the case. If you understand which abdominal sub-groups the exercises are intended to target, and have a rationale belief that your needs differ from the sequence showing – change the sequence. Generally speaking work from weakest to strongest in this phase.

Can I change the volume? Sure – but do you need to? I don't hesitate to say that this program is a generalization and therefore it is impossible for it to suit all. However, before you go and play with the variables, have a good hard think about the reasons that are driving you to change the program. Depending on what you are using abdominal training to achieve, I feel generally speaking that volume higher than that provided in this program is not needed.

For most of you, just do one set per exercise in Stage 1. For those who feel for whatever reason they want to do more volume, consider the second set on all or some of the exercises.

Can I change the reps? Sure. But again – do you need to? Review your driving force – is it rationale and objective? Have you given the parameters provided in this program adequate and objective trial?

Can I change the training method? The method recommended is basically a standard set approach – work set, rest, work set, rest etc. If you wanted to, and this is more applicable to those doing 2 sets on some or all of the exercises, you could use a circuit approach i.e. do one set on all without resting between exercises. Rest 1-2 minutes, then repeat the circuit. For whatever a (muscle) 'burn' will do for you, you will get it using this method!

Why abdominal exercises first in the workout? What I have brought to the world is the reality that if your abdominals are your weakest muscle group, or your priority – they should be done first! If you did have any concerns regarding residual fatigue, you could alter your exercise selection to minimize this. Keep in mind however my feelings that this fear is well... just another one of those unrealized fears most live their lives by! (One of my favorite authors, Denis Waitley, has an acronym for everything, including FEAR : False Evidence Appearing Real).

Does that mean I always suggest abs done first? NO! But if they are weaker than the rest of your body, if this weakness is increasing the risk of injury – then DO THEM FIRST! Generally speaking the reason I put them back in the program sequence (e.g. to the end) in the maximal strength phases of a program is to reduce the central nervous system (CNS) fatigue, saving for the bigger lifts.

What I have brought to the world is the reality that if your abdominals are your weakest muscle group, or your priority – they should be done first!

So in Stage 1 and 2, if you are lacking in the abdominal strength and control, I would expect the abs to appear first in the workout. In Stages 3 and 4, provided you have achieved your minimal abdominal standards, you could move them to the back of the workout. But you can and should be making this decision as you go based on the progress and standard you expect in your abdominal strength and control.

Recognize that each movement may progress at a different rate than another. What I am saying here is realize that the rate of change or improvement for any given exercise/action/muscle group may not be the same as another. For example, your lower abdominal drills may be improving slower than your upper abdominal drills. When this occurs, don't feel obliged to shift up to the next level of difficulty just because I have introduced the next stage. If you feel that the movement deserves a few more workouts or weeks to master it, don't move up to the next level of difficulty introduced in the new stage. On the other hand, you may feel that in other exercises you are ready go to the next level. Individualize your program in this way!

Does that mean I always suggest abs done first? NO!

Recommended Reference Material

Ian King's Guide To Abdominal Training – available at www.getbuffed.net

Chapter 10
The Control Drills

A small yet powerful addition!

Control drills by my definition include any exercises that focuses primarily on selective recruitment and quality of the movement, as opposed to the load lifted or reps performed That is, a qualitative focus rather than a quantitative focus.

They can be used to re-train a muscle, address muscle imbalances, or develop specific techniques (intra and inter muscular coordination). Therefore, the focuses is initially only on how well you do the movement. Rep and loading increments occur only when the technique can tolerate it, and remain much lower in the priorities of these types of exercises.

Control drills can and should form the bulk of the training program in the early stages of the program.

Control drills can and should form the bulk of the training program in the early stages of the program, and then be phased back to a maintenance role towards the end of the program.

When used in higher volume, such as the early stages of a training program, you may expect a higher degree of muscular fatigue. When used as in maintenance mode, there is no expectancy of muscular fatigue - more a 'switching on' of the muscles.

In this chapter I will discuss :

- Control Drills for Different Parts of the Body
- Guidelines for Control Drills
- Sample Control Drills for the Upper Body
- Sample Control Drills for the Lower Body

Control Drills for Different Parts of the Body

In the upper body, my major generalized focus in on scapula control and humeral positioning, through focus on the following movements :

In the trunk or mid-section of the body my major generalized focus is on abdominal and gluteal recruitment.

- Scapula depression (pulling the lower end of the shoulder blade or scapula down and in towards the spine).
- Scapula retraction (pulling the scapula in or medially towards the spine).
- External rotation of the humerus (rolling the upper arm outwards on its long axis i.e. with no movement in the upper arm).

In the lower body my major generalized focus is on hip positioning, femoral (upper leg) and patella (knee cap) control, through focus on the following movements :

- Increased tone and awareness of the 'lower abdominal' muscles.
- Posterior rotation of the pelvis through co-contraction of the gluteals and abdominals.
- Gluteal activation and control during extension of the femur, hip and trunk.
- Gluteal control during the external rotation of the femur.
- Activation of the vastus medialis oblique (VMO; the teardrop muscle above the knee on the inside of the thigh) specifically and quadriceps (quads) generally in knee stabilization.

In the trunk or mid-section of the body my major generalized focus is on abdominal and gluteal recruitment. I find that with most free weight/multi-joint based programs, the lower back receives adequate training. And provided the program has adequate hip dominant focus, the hamstrings and gluteals also get attention. I will address the mid-section control program in conjunction with the abdominal program in a later chapter.

Guidelines for Control Drills

The control drills should be performed with a focus on quality. You should use no or minimal external loading. Aim to maximize the strength of the contraction of the target muscles or the control of the movement or both.

Control drills should always come first in the workout. This will increase their contribution to selective muscle activation, which has both a performance enhancement and an injury prevention role.

Control drills should be performed all year round.

The average number of reps should be 10-20 reps per exercise. The speed of movement should always be controlled. There is little need for rest between sets of control drills.

The volume required from control drills influences the number of sets per drill. There will be times in the year when more than one set of each of the control drills is used, but for the most part, only one set of each should be performed.

Control drills should be performed all year round. The only variation will be in the volume, never the sequence within the workout.

Progression should be sought through improvements in the quality of contraction, the range through which the contraction can be maintained, and increased reps – in that order. Increase external load is an option but one that should be used sparingly. When you are performing controls drills for maintenance, which will be most of the year, do not necessarily look for progressive overload.

Another variable that can be manipulated is the number of exercises. In early stage programs, you may do a greater number of different control drills. In later stage programs, especially in maximal strength phases, you need only do 2-4 control drills.

Sample Control Drills for the Upper Body

Progression should be sought through improvements in the quality of contraction, the range through which the contraction can be maintained, and increased reps – in that order.

Flutters (for training of scapula retraction through rhomboids etc).
- Lie on your tummy.
- Hold arms out at 90 degrees to body.
- Raise and lower arms keeping perpendicular to body.
- Focus on squeezing shoulder blades together during the movement.
- Minimize the upper trap involvement.
- Use a 2-3 seconds up and same down.
- Don't touch ground with arms between reps but go very close.

Scarecrow (for training scapula depression through selective recruitment of the lower trapezius).
- Hold one hand up as if you are raising your hand to ask a question in a classroom, but bring the elbow down as low as you can whilst keeping the lower arm perpendicular to the ground and the arms in the frontal plane.
- Take the other arm up behind the body and place the back of your fingers on the shoulder blade of the side that has the arm in the air.
- Raise the arm in the air slowly, feeling for any movement of the scapula with the other hand behind the body.

- As soon as you feel and - and I mean any - scapula movement, terminate range, return to bottom position, reset and continue.
- When range ability starts to reduce, terminate set.

Side Lying External Dumbbell (DB) Rotation.
- Lie on your side on the ground.
- Place the top side elbow beside the body and have the elbow bent to 90 degrees.
- Hold a very light dumbbell (DB) in this hand and without the elbow moving at all from the top of the body, raise and lower the DB, keeping the elbow at 90 degrees.

Prone Limited Range DB Row.
- Lie face down on a prone bench, arms off each side of the bench.
- Hold a DB in each hand.
- The position of the arms (i.e. prone, supine or neutral) can be varied.
- Row the DBs by lifting the elbows up as high as they can go, then lower the DBs down about 1/3 of the way down. This is the range you will be using – the top 1/3 of the full movement.

Increase external load is an option but one that should be used sparingly.

Sample Control Drills for the Lower Body

Light leg extensions (for raising patella-femoral joint temperature/lubrication and rehearsing co-contraction of hamstring and quadriceps).

- Perform one legged-leg extensions, completing on reps on one leg before going to other side.
- Place the hand from the opposite side on the VMO (the tear-drop muscle just above the knee on the inside – aim to contract it as much as possible, feeling for the tension that this generates in this muscle.
- Contract the hamstring on the same side at the same time.

Prone lying single leg hip / thigh extensions (for raising gluteal / hamstring firing).

- Lie face down on a bench or Roman Chair (if using a bench, the higher the better).
- Extend one leg up till it is straight in line with trunk and then lower it down, stopping before the foot touches the ground. Focus on the gluteals and hamstrings doing the work, in that order.
- Once all reps are completed, perform set on other leg.

Side Lying Lateral Leg Raise (for raising the recruitment of the gluteals).

- Lie on your side on the ground.
- Raise one leg up laterally (to the side) to about 45 degrees, keep the long axis of the foot parallel to the ground.
- Lower back down, stopping before the foot touches the ground. Repeat.
- Focus on the higher section of your gluteals to perform this movement.
- Once all reps are completed, perform set on other leg.

Co-Contraction Lunge.

- Stand in static lunge position i.e. one leg in front of the other, in a long wide stance.
- Place the opposite hand to the lead side leg on the VMO of the lead leg.
- Place the hand from the same side as the lead leg on the upper gluteals.
- Use this hand contact to encourage higher level muscle firing from these two muscles.
- Lower the hips only about 1/3 of the range available, and then come back up to the top of the movement but stop short of lockout.
- Once all reps are completed, perform set on other leg.

Lying Supine Single Leg Hip/Thigh Extension.

- Lie on your back on the ground.
- Bend one leg up till the knee is 90 degrees, with that foot flat.

When you are performing controls drills for maintenance, which will be most of the year, do not necessarily look for progressive overload.

- Keep the other leg straight out on the ground.
- Put your weight through that foot and raise the straight leg up till the straight leg is in line with the thigh of the bent knee, and there is a straight line between the shoulders and the knee.
- Lower back down but do not rest fully on the ground.
- Once all reps are completed, perform set on other leg.

Assisted Squat (to prepare the joints and tissue for the range of movement in the squat).
- Hold onto a vertical frame with both hands.
- Taking a lot of weight through the hands, lower down about 1/10 of the range you will use in the squat.
- Use the hands maximally to return to the top but avoid full lockout.
- Do 9 more reps, and in each subsequent rep increase the range and reduce the work of the arms progressively
- The final rep, rep 10, should see you using the range you will use in the workout, with minimal effort by the hands.

Another variable that can be manipulated is number of exercises. In early stage programs, you may be more different control drills.

Recommended Reference Material

Ian King's Guide To Control Drills – available at www.getbuffed.net
How To Teach Strength Training Exercises Video - available at www.kingsports.net

Chapter 11

The Get Buffed!™ II Workout : Get More Buffed!

A level up from the original one!

You can and should make the individual adjustments you want based on the guidelines provided earlier in the book.

The programs will be presented as follows, in four stages. Remember you can and should make the individual adjustments you want based on the guidelines provided earlier in the book in the 'Designing the Workout' chapter.

- ❑ Stage One
- ❑ Stage Two
- ❑ Stage Three
- ❑ Stage Four

Within each stage, there are the three loading options :

- o Hypertrophy/Lower Training Age
- o Hypertrophy-neural/Intermediate Training Age
- o Neural/Advanced Training Age

The *Get Buffed!™* II (Get More Bufffed!) programs are based on a four day a week (4/wk) split routine. The general intent of the program is for the workouts to occur as per the following table :

Table 20 – General layout of workouts for this program.

Sun.	Mon.	Tue.	Wed.	Thu.	Fri.	Sat.
	Part A	Part B	Optional 'Fat Burning' Workout; Stretching Session	Part C	Part D	Optional 'Fat Burning' Workout; Stretching Session

The Optional 'Fat Burning Workouts' would consist of 20-40 minutes of low intensity general activity such as walking, jogging, cycling or similar. The Stretching sessions on these same days would consist of 40-90 minutes of focused stretching. The specific parameters of these two activities, the 'Fat Burning' and Stretching Session, would be influenced by your specific needs and goals at the time. For a further discussion on these, refer to the related chapters in this book.

Each workout will involve the following components :

- Warm up
- Stretching
- Abdominal Training
- Control Drills
- Body of the Workout

This is the recommended order for at least Stages 1 and 2. You may see, in Stages 3 and 4, an altering of the sequencing of abdominal training, as shown below, but that is ONLY if you are satisfied with the strength of your abdominals relative to the remainder of the body.

- Warm up
- Stretching
- Control Drills
- Body of the Workout
- Abdominal Training

Note the only difference between the two workout sequences shown above is the placement of the abdominals exercises in the sequence.

The discussion of variables relating to these components are contained in the prior chapters. The description of how to perform the various exercises are provided after the workouts, with the exception of the stretching and control drills. The exercise descriptions for these are provided in the earlier chapters of the same name.

In the next few pages I have provided a brief refresher on notes and background information you may need to interpret and perform these workouts.

The Optional 'Fat Burning Workouts' would consist of 20-40 minutes of low intensity general activity such as walking, jogging, cycling or similar.

Recommended Reference Material

The *Get Buffed!*™ **Program Video Series** – available at www.getbuffed.net
The *How To Write Strength Training Programs* book – available at www.kingsports.net.

Notes Supporting The Workouts

Here are some **codes** that you will see used in the program :

Load and reps and rest
BW = bodyweight; EXT = external load; ECC = eccentric overload
AMRAP or AMRP= as many reps as possible
RP or R/Per = rest period; ALT = alternate with another exercise

Body relative to bar or equipment
B = back or behind; F = front or to the front

Grips
WG = wide grip; MG = medium grip; CG = close grip; RG = reverse grip

Stances
WS = wide stance; MS = medium stance; NS = narrow stance

Bar Position/Lines of Movement
HB = in the squat, sit the bar high on the back/neck; in the bench press lower the bar high up on chest (to neck);
MB = in the squat, sit the bar in a medium position on the back; in the bench press, lower the bar to the middle of the chest;
LB = in the squat, sit the bar in a low position on the back/neck; in the bench press, lower the bar low on the chest;

Foot Positions
FA = feet up in the air (e.g. in bench press); FB = feet on bench; FD = feet down on the ground

Weight or Body Position relative to the support base
OG = plates start on the ground; OB = plates start on blocks; SOB = you stand on a block

Other Positions
Prone = face down or palm down
Supine=face up or palm up

Equipment
EZ = ezy curl bar; DB = dumbbell

Here is further **background information** that you may need. You will find more detail on this in the original *Get Buffed!*™ book :

Speed of Movement

- If speed indicators are given, the first number refers to the lowering (eccentric phase) speed in seconds, the middle (second) number to the duration of the pause in seconds, and the last number (third) to the duration of the lifting (concentric phase) in seconds. For example, 804 = 8 second lowering time, no pause, and 4 second lifting time.
- The majority of movements are to performed with a controlled lowering, pause, and then an explosive lift - unless otherwise indicated, think "quick" and try to lift "quickly", with speed.
- A 1 as the third number means you should be trying to lift (concentric phase) explosively. As fast as you can. However it may not look fast. When an asterisk (*) appears as the third number, or as any number, you should be trying to also be as explosive as possible – but this must look fast also! Which may mean less load than if it were a '1' as a third number.
- The warm-ups reps are in most instances to be performed at a normal speed i.e. 311.
- Olympic-type movements, emphasis should be placed on the speed of the movement, rather than the amount lifted.

Variations of Speeds

There will be times when the conventional speeds are replaced or supplemented by unique movement speeds or patterns and these include :

- **1 1/2s or 1.5s in pushing movements** (e.g. bench press, squat) = Lower down to the bottom of your range, pause, then come up 1/3 –1/2 of the way, pause, then go back down to the bottom, pause, then come up all the way. This is one rep. Avoid full lockout. Pause, and repeat.
- **1 1/2s or 1.5s in pulling movements** (e.g. chin ups, leg curls) = Lift all the way up to the top of your range, pause, then come down 1/3 – 1/2 of the way, pause, then go back up to the top, pause, then lower down all the way. This is one rep. Allow full stretch. Pause, and repeat.
- **3 x 3** = This would require you to stop three times during the eccentric phase, for three seconds each time. Vary the stopping positions.

Warm Up Sets

- When only one number appears in the warm-up (WU) column a weight approximately 50 - 60% of the weight you intend using in the work sets is to be used at the number of reps indicated.
- When two numbers appear in the warm-up (WU) column the first set of reps are to be performed at a weight of approximately 40% of the intended work weight and the second set at approximately 70% of the intended work weight.
- When three numbers appear in the warm-up column (WU) they are to be performed at approximately 40% (first WU set), 60% (second WU set) and 80% (third WU set) of the intended work weight.
- If a warm down set is indicated, and if the lightest bar/load in the gym for that exercise causes you fatigue in the warm up set, it just became the work-set and move on to the next exercise.

Rest Periods

- Note that the rest periods may change from stage to stage.
- Use only the full rest period if required - ensure full recovery prior to starting next set.
- The rest period indicated does not need to be taken in full between warm up sets.
- If there is a great discrepancy between the rest period indicated and the rest period you feel you need there may be a problem with your training approach - consult your instructor.

Weight Selection

- Select a weight in the first week that allows you perform the prescribed sets and reps with correct technique.
- Increase the weights in small increments each week on every exercise if possible.
- If you remain on the same weight and reps for more than two consecutive weeks there may be a problem in your weight selection which requires modifying.
- Never sacrifice correct technique or safety in an attempt to lift heavier weight - each person has a technique limit on each of their exercises which if they exceed they will not be able to perform the exercise in the prescribed manner.

Safety and Spotting

- When the bar is above the body e.g. in the bench press, do not hesitate to use a spotter in the event that you can not complete the movement.
- Minimize the use of 'assisted reps' i.e. where your spotter helps you up and then you continue to lower the bar again, he helps you up, etc.
- Use common sense to avoid injury, etc. if it hurts - stop.

Stage 1

Stage 1 - Overview

In Stage 1 (and Stage 2) the lower body dominates over the upper body if you use a linear periodization, and in Stage 1 and 3 if you use an alternating approach. In Stage 1 upper body pulling dominates over upper body pushing. You do all your pulling in the first upper body workout of the week and all your pushing in the second or latter workout of the week.

Now historically it is nothing new to split pushing and pulling in strength training, although I don't use this method as much as it has been used historically. But what I am doing that is less conventional is the sequencing of priority from pulling to pushing. Not many programs get the pushing done later in the week. Why generalize - ask yourself - how many programs have you left bench and shoulder press to later in the week? And you are wondering why you have got a muscle imbalance!?!

How long would you have to prioritize your weaknesses before your muscle imbalances are corrected? One way to answer this is to simply determine how long (in say months or years) you previously trained in an unbalanced way - and in rough terms you can expect somewhere between half that time and that same amount of time spent prioritizing your weaknesses. Not the answer you wanted to hear I know! However that is worst case. With smarter programming, you can reduce this time.

So what's in store in Stage 1?

The **abdominal program** in this stage generally speaking is injury prevention focused. I feel that the primary purpose of abdominal training is to contribute to the health of the lower back, hips and lower extremities. I placed sport transfer second because of the general transfer this program may have. There is no attempt to be sport specific or hyper-specific in the program.

In the **lower body program** in this stage I propose a hip dominant priority over quad dominant. By this I mean we are going to do deadlift and deadlift variations early in the training week, and squat and squat variations later in the training week. I will then return this back to 'normal' in Stages 3 and 4. Why do I suggest starting out with hip dominant exercises as a priority in the training week over quad dominant exercises in this stage? Because I have observed a pattern of quad dominance in the traditional and typical mainstream training programs. Chances are you have prioritized quad dominant exercises to a greater extent than hip dominant exercises in your training history!

In the **upper body program** in this stage I have given priority to what I have observed is most strength training participants greatest weaknesses – their pulling muscles, or more specifically their ability to pull in horizontal (scapula retract) and vertical (scapula depress) planes. Additionally, arms are prioritized over the core pushing/pulling muscles in Stage 1. Within the pulling in Stage 1, I have prioritized horizontal pull over vertical pull and in the pushing, vertical pushing over horizontal pushing. Simply based on my experience and observations of common muscle imbalances.

The following provides **general information about this stage of the program**:

A tri-set is intended to be done as follows : one set of the first exercise, 0-10sec rest, then one set of the second exercise, 0-10sec rest, then one set of the third exercise. If there is a warm up and a work set involved, or more than one work set, this cycle is repeated after resting up to 2-4 minutes (e.g. 2 minutes for hyper/intro version, 3 minutes for mixed hyper-neural/intermediate version, and 4 minutes for neural/advanced version).

As a general guide use less rest between sets during the tri-set and between cycles of the tri-set in week one, and you can allow more rest time to be added each subsequent week of the stage provided you don't exceed the time frames shown.

Now go and *Get Buffed!*™

Stage 1 – Warm Up / Stretching / Abdominal / Control Drills

A & C Day

Exercise	Warm up	Work	Speed	Rest
Warm Up		10-20 minutes of light aerobic type activity e.g. stationary bike		
Stretch		20-40 minutes of lower body stretching		
Abdominals				
Thin tummy variations	nil	1-2x10	313 or 5 sec holds	0-30s
Toes to sky	nil	1-2x10	313 or 5 sec holds	0-30s
Side raises on ground	nil	1-2x10-20	313 per side	0-30s
Side lying trunk and leg raises	nil	1-2x5-10	3-5s holds Or 313	0-30s
Seated thin tummy/squeeze cheeks	1x5-10		5s holds	0-30s
Control Drills				
Light leg extensions	nil	2x15-20	202	0-30s
Prone lying single leg hip / thigh extensions	nil	2x15-30	202	0-30s
Side Lying Lateral Leg Raise	nil	2x15-30	202	0-30s
Co-Contraction Lunge	nil	2x10-20	202	0-30s
Lying Supine Single Leg Hip/Thigh Extension	nil	2x5-20	202	0-30s
Assisted Squat	nil	1x10	202	0-30s
Workout				

Stage 1 : A & C Day – Abdominal Exercise Descriptions

Here are descriptions of the abdominal exercises involved in A and C day, Stage 1 of the *Get Buffed!*™ II (Get More Buffed!) four (4) stage program.

Thin Tummy Variations : The 'thin tummy drill' is the corner stone I build my abdominal programs upon, yet it is one of the hardest to learn.

Lie on your back, knee bent, feet flat, place both hands under your belt line, with your fingers heading down into the pubic area and the thumbs placed higher up on the rectus abdominus (upper abdominal region); throughout all the following levels of difficulty, use the fingers to provide feedback that the 'lower abdominals' (obliques and transverse abdominus) are contracted, pulling the lower tummy thinner and creating a high level of tension under the skin; and that the upper abdominal region is hollowed, and non-contracted; and that this relationship is held. Should it at any time change or you feel that it is going to change e.g. upper tummy bulge, pelvis anteriorly rotate, terminate the range or the set. I focus more on how the muscles are 'set' than on the pressure of lumbar to ground or position of pelvis, although both are symptomatic of a good 'set' position.

Initially you may struggle to even find the muscles I want you to contract! Work with 5-second holds, 10 reps a set, and the next step is to be able to breath normally during the isometric contractions!

I have at least five levels of difficulty that I teach and this simple isometric contraction is level one. In Stage 1 you should be happy to master Level 1 and maybe progress to Level 2.

Level 1 - isometric holds (looking for above 'set' position) in the lying, knee bent positions.

Level 2 - as above, but lift one leg up, lower it, reset, other leg etc.

Level 3 - as above, but when you lift one leg up, extend it out towards the ground as far as you can control the hip position and abdominal shape (i.e. the 'set' position).

Level 4 - as above, but start with both knees up, bent to 90 degrees knees and hips, cycling one leg out towards a parallel to ground position at a time as far as 'set' position control allows.

Level 5 - as above, but extending both legs out together.

Notes :

Speed of movement – isometric holds for 5-10 seconds; dynamic movements at 313. For an explanation of these speed timings and how to interpret them, refer to the original *Get Buffed!*™ book. Basically, the first number is the time in seconds to complete the eccentric or lowering phase of the lift; the middle number is the pause at each end in seconds; and the third number is the time in seconds to complete the concentric or lifting phase.

Selecting appropriate level - the only way to really know what level of difficulty is appropriate is to perform a rep or two at each level, starting from the least difficult, until it appears that you are being challenged. I call this trial and error! Do not continue on looking for failure – work with a level that is manageable. In this exercise you really need to educate yourself to feel for when they lose the 'set' position.

Toes to Sky : This exercise is a bit easier to teach. It is not as 'fine' in its requirements, but can still be misinterpreted. Lie on your back, arms out on the ground at 90 degrees to the trunk, have your legs together, 90 degrees hip flexion, so that legs are vertical.

I identify at least three levels of difficulty in this drill, but don't expect you to go beyond level 1 in Stage 1.

Level 1 - lift the pelvis as far off the ground whilst maintaining a totally vertical leg position (initially this may not be very far at all, at even in the most competent person, the movement range is limited to a few inches) and hold for 5-10 seconds.

Level 2 - as above, but bend one knee to 90 degrees at the knee; alternate each rep which leg is bent, which is straight.

Level 3 - as above, but bend both knees so that the knees are bent to 90 degrees.

Notes :

Speed of movement – A controlled lift, a steady hold for 5-10 seconds, a controlled lower; no use of momentum, keeping legs (or upper leg at least) always totally vertical.

Arm positions - Keep arms out to side on ground, 90 degrees to trunk.

Selecting appropriate level – Trial and error.

Side Raises on Ground : These are my basic exercise for developing lateral trunk flexion. Whilst it can be argued that the position and action is not totally isolated to flexion in the horizontal plane, it is a low level exercise appropriate for the first quality of strength - control and stability.

Description - Lie on your back, knees bent to about 90 degrees, and knees together. Roll the knees over together so that they are on the ground, with the shoulders and upper back still parallel to the ground. Now flex the trunk, basically up towards the roof or sky. I like to have the fingers lightly touching the front of the head, elbows out at 45 degrees from the body, and arm/elbow angle not changing during the lift. The placement of the hands will alter the level of difficulty.

The further the hands are above the head, the harder the movement.

Notes :

Speed of movement – Controlled movements at 313.

Arm positions – Provided above.

Selecting appropriate level – Trial and error.

Side Lying Trunk and Leg Raises : This is an additional lateral flexion exercise, one that includes both trunk and hip/thigh lateral flexion. This is a fairly unique exercise. Lie on your side on the ground, with your hands straight out either side of your head, in line with your body, and legs straight. You must start on your side and stay on our side. You can lock your hands together if you want. Now simultaneously raise your arms and your legs so that neither of the lower arm or leg are in contact with the ground.

Notes :

Speed of movement – Your have a choice of a 3-5 sec hold in the top position or a controlled movement of 313.

Arm positions - You can lock your hands together if you want.

Selecting appropriate level – If you are struggling with balance you may find one or the other speed option easier, but there is not a lot of difference in which one you use.

Seated Thin Tummy/squeeze Cheeks : This is an exercise from the category I describe as 'co-contractions of the abs and gluts'. They appear to be a very benign exercise and are relatively simple. Don't underestimate their contribution however!

Sit on the end of a prone bench with your knees and feet together, feet on the ground, chest up and back straight. Now create that thin dish abdominal position I described in the thin tummy drill – make the lower abdominals thin and contract the lower abdominals. You can use your hands down on your abs in the same way for feedback on the quality of this contraction. Now also squeeze your cheeks in a manner that results in you 'levitating' a inch or so off the bench! You may find that sucking up the pelvic floor contributes to the quality of the contraction!

Notes :

Speed of movement – use of 5 sec hold in the top.

Arm positions – In your abdominal region, getting feedback (same as for thin tummy drill).

Selecting appropriate level – just the one! If you found this too easy, you could do the same thing standing.

Stage 1 – Warm Up / Stretching / Abdominal / Control Drills

B & D Day

Exercise	Warm up	Work	Speed	Rest
Warm Up	optional 5-15 minutes of light aerobic type activity e.g. stationary bike			
Stretch	10-20 minutes of upper body stretching			
Abdominals				
Slow up/slow down (or cheat up/slow lower)	nil	1-2x10 or 5-15 sec lowers if using alternative	515	0-30s
Reverse curl downs	nil	1-2x10	101,202,303 etc.	0-30s
Russian twist with leg cycle in V-sit	nil	1-2x15-30 full rotations	202 -303	0-30s
Lateral leg lowers	nil	1-2x10-20 full rotations	303	0-30s
Push up position on knees	nil	1x5-15	5s holds	0-30s
Control Drills				
Flutters	nil	2x10-20	202	0-30s
Scarecrow	nil	2x 5-15	202	0-30s
Side Lying Ext DB Rotation	nil	2x10-20	202	0-30s
Prone Limited Range DB Row	nil	2x10-20	202	0-30s

Workout

Stage 1 : B & D Day – Abdominal Exercise Descriptions

Here are descriptions of the abdominal exercises involved in B and D day, Stage 1 of the *Get Buffed!* ™ II (Get More Buffed!) four (4) stage program.

Slow Up/Slow Down : These are my core exercise for developing trunk flexion. In Stage 1 I have nominated specifically the slow up/slow down drill, or the cheat up/slow lower - which as you will see below are two of the five levels of difficulty I provide in this cornerstone trunk flexion drill. It allows excellent progression for all levels of competence – from those who cannot sit up at all through to those who can sit up using the most difficult variations. The basic position for this exercise is lying on the back, knees bent to about 90 degrees, and feet flat on the floor. Your feet are not to be anchored under anything. Then you sit up or curl up the trunk, in most part to a full sitting position.

The exception to this is when I say 'cheat up'. In this case, go from lying on the ground with your knees bent to 90 degrees, feet flat, to sitting up fully – anyhow you can. For example, you may want to throw your hands from over your head to in front of you at the time of sitting up, to make it possible. This variation is for those who cannot complete a controlled, slow speed sit-up (the concentric phase).

<u>Control progressions</u>

Cheat ups / slow down

Cheat ups / slow down + isometric stops during lower

Reverse curl downs

Slow up / slow down

Slow up / slow downs with isometric pauses during the up phase

Notes :

Speed of movement – It is critical in these control exercises that the time indicated for each contraction phase is evenly distributed throughout the movement i.e. no momentum or acceleration is to be used during the concentric phase, and no collapsing during lower phase; if momentum or acceleration is used during the concentric phase, a lower level of difficulty is recommended; if collapsing occurs during lower phase, use a shorter total time for the lowering, with the aim to allow a uniform quicker movement throughout the eccentric.

Arm positions - Each of these levels of difficulty have at least 5 different arm positions that provide further variety/levels of difficulty.

1 = arms remain parallel to ground, pointed towards feet.

2 = upper arms remain parallel to ground, hands on opposite elbow.

3 = upper arms remain parallel to ground, hands on opposite shoulder.

4 = hands touching forehead, elbows out at 45 degrees to front of head.

5 = hands touching side of head, elbows forming a straight line either side.

Selecting appropriate level - Trial and error.

Reverse Curl-Downs : These are actually a progression in the above exercise, but I am going to get you to do this as an additional exercise in this program. Lie on the ground on your back, and bend your knees to about 90 degrees, with your feet flat on the floor. Your feet are not to be anchored under anything. Start in the full setup position, with arms parallel to ground. The arm position can be varied to alter load (i.e. make it harder) if needed. Lower your trunk back to the ground an inch or two, counting 'one thousand and one' (one second) as you complete the lowering, then take that same time to return back to the top starting position. Do both in a controlled, non-accelerated manner. Then lower your trunk back towards the ground again this time going a few more inches, basically the range involved as you count to one thousand and one, two-thousand and two (two seconds). Then return back to the top starting position in this same time frame. Repeat this method adding a second each rep, and going a bit further down each time.

Basically, if you are able to do your final and tenth rep all the way down to the ground, and control back to the top position in the same non-accelerated manner, you would divide range into ten equal points, each point being the point to which you lower to each subsequent rep. However if you are not able to either lower under control in 10 seconds all the way down, or return back up in this controlled manner in 10 seconds, and without your feet moving, then you need to identify a point just above the angle at which you collapse, and this will be your range for the 10th rep. Then create 10 equal points from the top, seated position to this trunk angle, and these will be your end-points for each of the 10 reps.

Notes :

Speed of movement – It is critical in these control exercises that the time indicated for each contraction phase is evenly distributed throughout the movement i.e. no momentum or acceleration is to use during the concentric phase, and no collapsing during lower phase; so only use a range that allows this, and divide it into 10 levels, one for each rep.

Arm positions - Each of these levels of difficulty have at least 5 different arm positions that provide further variety/levels of difficulty. They are the same as the ones described in the slow up/slow down exercise.

Selecting appropriate level – Use trial and error. If you find you are not able to perform a certain range at a rep prior to the 10th rep, this rep becomes the 10 rep in future.

Russian Twist with Leg Cycle in V-sit : This is a core option in the trunk rotation category. Sit on the ground, and lean the trunk back to about 45 degrees. Take your feet off the ground, and have one knee brought up to your chest and the other leg out in front, parallel but not resting on the ground (just like you were cycling with the legs!)

Now rotate your body to one side, rotating from the waist. If the base of the waist stops rotating, don't look to rotate the upper trunk further. At the same time lower the bent leg down to nearly straight and parallel but not touching the ground as you bring the other knee up. This leg position swap and the trunk rotation should happen simultaneously. For coordination, try bringing the knee up on the side that you are rotating the trunk towards.

Notes :

Speed of movement – Use a controlled two to three seconds to one side and two to three seconds back to the other side. The legs swap and cycle in this same controlled manner.

Arm positions - Place your hands out in front at 90 degrees to the body, interlocking thumbs gently.

Lateral Leg Lowers : This is a rotation drill for the hips and legs. Lie on your back, legs in the air together, and arms out at 90 degrees to the body. Keep the head down on the ground also. Now lower the legs to one side, going all the way down to but not resting on the ground, maintaining that 90 degree angle between legs and upper body. Keep the upper body still, head included, at all times.

Now return the legs back up to the vertical and over to the other side in the same way.

Notes :

Speed of movement – Use a controlled three seconds to one side and three seconds back to the other side.

Arm positions - Place your arms out at 90 degrees to the body, resting on the ground.

Push Up Position on knees : This is a core drill for the category I call integration. I don't get carried away with advanced options in this category until I have raised the abilities in the above categories.

Lie on the ground on your stomach, legs out straight and together and arms under the chest. Have the lower arms parallel to each other and a few inches apart under the chest. Now raise the body onto the knees and elbows, or the feet and elbows, depending upon the level of difficulty you want. Raise to and hold in a position where the knee or ankle (depending upon which option you chose) to the shoulders is a straight line, but not necessarily parallel to the ground. After the hold duration, lower back down to the start position i.e. between each rep.

Notes :

Speed of movement – Hold the top position for five seconds. Recover for 1-2 seconds at the bottom position (resting on ground).

Arm positions - Have the lower arms parallel to each other and a few inches apart under the chest (knee or toe option). If you are using the full pushup option, go with the arms in a typical push up position. Levels of difficulty include :

1 = Raise to elbows and knees

2 = Raise to elbows and toes

3 = Raise to hands and toes (full push up position)

Stage 1, Option 1 - Hypertrophy / Lower Training Age

A Day

Exercise	Warm up	Work	Speed	Rest
Shrugs Tri-set				
1.Very wide grip, barbell	10	6-8+	311	tri-set
2.Medium grip, barbell	10	8-10+	311	tri-set
3.Medium, underhand grip, barbell (option with DBs)	10	10-12	311	tri-set
Thigh abduction (single or double)	10	6-8+ 8-10+ 10-12	311	strip set
Prone Hip/thigh extension (single or double)	10	10+10+10	311	strip set
Good morning (single or double)	10	10	1.5	½-1m
Stiff legged deadlift (single or double)	nil	10	3x3	½-1m
King deadlift	nil	1xmax reps	311	1-2m
Deadlift – WG/OG	nil	10	3x3	1-2m
1 and a quarter deadlifts-WG	nil	10	1.3	1-2m
Snatch Pulls OG/WG	8	8	10*	1-2m

Stage 1, Option 2 - Hypertrophy-neural / Intermediate Training Age

A Day

Exercise	Warm up	Work	Speed	Rest
Shrugs Tri-set				
1.Medium, under-hand grip, barbell	10	4-6+	311	tri-set
2.Medium grip, barbell	10	6-8+	311	tri-set
3.Very wide grip, barbell (option with DBs)	10	8-10	311	tri-set
Thigh abduction (single or double)	10	4-6+ 6-8+ 8-10	311	strip set
Hip/thigh extension (single or double)	10	8+8+8	311	strip set
Good morning (single or double)	8	8	1.5	1m
Stiff legged deadlift (single or double)	nil	8	3x3	1m
King deadlift	nil	1xmax reps	311	1-2m
Deadlift – WG/OG 3x3	nil	8	3x3	2m
1 and a quarter deadlifts-WG	nil	8	1.3	2m
Snatch Pulls OG/WG	6	6	10*	2m

Stage 1, Option 3 - Neural/Advanced Training Age

A Day

Exercise	Warm up	Work	Speed	Rest
Deadlift (WG/OG/ 3x3)	nil	8	3x3	2m
1 and a quarter (deadlifts-WG)	nil	8	1.3	2m
Snatch Pulls -OG/WG	6	6	10*	2m
King deadlift	nil	1xmax reps	311	1-2m
Stiff legged deadlift (single or double)	nil	8	3x3	1m
Good morning (single or double)	8	8	1.5	1m
Hip/thigh extension (single or double)	8	8+8+8	311	strip set
Thigh abduction (single or double)	10	4-6+ 6-8+ 8-10	311	strip set
Shrugs Tri-set				
1.Medium, underhand (grip, barbell)	10	4-6+	311	tri-set
2.Medium grip, barbell	10	6-8+	311	tri-set
3.Very wide grip, barbell (option with DBs)	10	8-10	311	tri-set

Stage 1 : A Day - Exercise Descriptions

Here are descriptions of the exercises involved in A day, Stage 1 of the *Get Buffed!* ™ II (Get More Buffed!) four (4) stage program.

Shrug Tri-set : This involves three variations of shrugs. Use a barbell unless you have a bilateral imbalance, in which case use DB on all except the wide grip option. The order of the three variations is dependant upon which program you are using. Remember to keep your elbows locked out throughout the movement, keep the head vertically aligned but pulling the chin in, and push the chest up. The use of straps is not recommended for the hypertrophy option, optional in the hypertrophy-neural option, and probably needed in the neural option.

Thigh Abduction : I know – you may think it is a silly little exercise. Just do it! And focus on the recruitment of the gluts whilst doing it – this is more important than the load used. You can do the leg abduction (taking leg away) either on a dedicated machine, or low pulley cable, or even lying on your side on the ground with ankle weights. Keep the foot orientation neutral (not turned in, not turned out) during the movement. To exploit the strip set concept – go to fatigue within the rep bracket indicated, rest only as long as it takes to reduce the load to one that allows you to achieve the reps within the next rep bracket indicated, repeat for a third set. You will need more external loading the lower in reps you choose to do.

Hip/Thigh Extension : Again, you decide whether you do this one single or double leg based on your bilateral balance. Lie on your tummy on a prone bench (preferably one that is higher than standard) or on a device dedicated to this lift. Have your trunk fully supported, with your legs off. Extend your leg/s from just off the floor to in line with the trunk, focusing on squeezing the gluts. Again, focus more on recruitment than loading (i.e. feel for it in the gluts and hamstrings), and keep the foot orientation neutral during the extension in particular. You will need external loading for the lower reps if you chose to use the more advanced loading parameters.

Good Morning : Stand on one or two legs (your decision) - with a bar on the shoulders, with the knees only slightly bent, flex forward at the waist until your head (ideally) is near you knee), using a rounded back technique, and then stand back up again. Do not allow the knee angle to change during the lift. This lift is done using the 1 ½ technique i.e. go all the way down, pause, come up half way, pause, go back down all the way, pause, then return to the starting position - this is one rep! If doing the one leg version, have the other foot off the ground, but kept roughly parallel with the leg doing the supporting.

Stiff Legged Deadlift : Again, choose between the single or double leg versions. The technique for this lift is as per the Good Morning. If doing the single leg, hold a DB in each hand. If using the double leg, hold a barbell with both hands, using a medium width prone grip. The difference from the Good Morning will be this – I want you to use the chest up, butt out, flat back technique. Only go down as far as you can whilst keeping the hips and spine aligned.

King Deadlift : This is a single leg bent knee deadlift. Stand on one leg (starting with the weak side) and bend the other leg up until the lower leg is parallel to the ground. Hands on hips or by side. The aim is to bend the knee of the supporting leg until the knee of the non-supporting leg is brushing the ground. In reality, you may have to settle for a shorter range (you'll understand why I say this as soon as you do this workout). If this is the case - and I expect it will be - look to increase the range from workout to workout.

You are allowed to flex (bend) forward at the waist as much as you want, and doing so will increase the gluteal involvement. Keep the working knee aligned neutrally (e.g.

over the middle of the foot) throughout the movement. Take 3 seconds to lower, 1 second pause each end and 2 seconds to lift. No warm up set needed. When you can do more than 15-20 reps FULL RANGE look to hold DBs in the hands.

Snatch Pulls – WG : The snatch pull is a wide grip deadlift to above the knees, and then accelerating to the toes and simultaneously shrugging your shoulders in the top position. If you struggle with the wider grip, use a medium, just outside shoulders grip (clean pull). Basically the technique is as per the deadlift except for the more aggressive acceleration in the second pull. The criteria for load selection in addition to trunk/hip/scapula technique, is the height and speed of the pull (on toes and traps). Avoid any elbow flexion until the last moment, at which time allow the bar to rise if the acceleration has been significant.

1 ¼ Deadlifts - WG: This is my standard wide grip deadlift technique (which I will outline in the next exercise description. The difference here is that once the bar is just above the knees, pause, lower back down to just below the knees, pause, then stand up fully before returning to rest the bar on the ground. This is one rep.

Deadlifts - WG : Using a wide grip, and starting from the bottom position, weight rested on the ground. Switch on the primary stabilizers before take off – the abdominals, gluteals, upper back, and extend the legs to take up the slack before take off. On the way up, stop three (3) times, for three (3) seconds each time. Vary the points at which you are stopping, and spread these stopping points out over the full range. Lower the bar 'normally' i.e. not isometric stops during lowering. Remember, If you are experiencing lower back pain or excessive fatigue, you are using a technique different to what I recommend.

Stage 1, Option 1 – Hypertrophy / Lower Training Age

B Day

Exercise	Warm up	Work	Speed	Rest
Forearm Flexion	10	8-10+	311	tri-set
(1 or 2 arm)		10-12+	311	i.e. { }
		12-15	311	or <=10s
Bicep Tri-set :				
Incline DB Curl	10	10-12+	311	tri-set
Reverse Curl EZ	10	8-10+	311	i.e. { }
on PB				or <=10s
Seated Hammer	10	6-8	311	
DB C+T				
Horizontal Pull Tri-set:				
Prone DB Fly	10	10-12+	311	tri-set
Bent Over Row	10	8-10+	311	i.e. { }
(WG/HB)				or <=10s
Seated Row	10	6-8	311	
(U/hand grip)				
Vertical Pull Tri-set:				
DB Pullover	10	10-12+	311	tri-set
Lat Pulldown-WG/B	10	8-10+	311	i.e. { }
Chin up	10	6-8	311	or <=10s
(palm facing you)				

Stage 1, Option 2 - Hypertrophy-neural / Intermediate Training Age

B Day

Exercise	Warm up	Work	Speed	Rest
Forearm Flexion	10	6-8+	311	tri-set
(1 or 2 arm)		8-10+	311	i.e. { }
		10-12	311	or <=10s
Bicep Tri-set :				
Incline DB Curl	10	8-10+	311	tri-set
Reverse Curl	10	6-8+	311	i.e. { }
(EZ on PB)				or <=10s
Seated Hammer	10	4-6	311	
DB Curl+Twist				
Horizontal Pull Tri-set:				
Prone DB Fly	10	8-10+	311	tri-set
Bent Over Row	10	6-8+	311	i.e. { }
(WG/HB)				or <=10s
Seated Row	10	4-6	311	
(U/hand grip)				
Vertical Pull Tri-set:				
DB Pullover	10	8-10+	311	tri-set
Lat Pulldown	10	6-8+	311	i.e. { }
(WG/B)				or <=10s
Chin up	10	4-6	311	
(palm facing you)				

Stage 1, Option 3 - Neural/Advanced Training Age

B Day

Exercise	Warm up	Work	Speed	Rest
Forearm Flexion	10	6-8+	311	tri-set
(1 or 2 arm)		8-10+	311	i.e. { }
		10-12	311	or <=10s
Bicep Tri-set :				
Seated Hammer	10	4-6+	311	tri-set
DB C+T				i.e. { }
Reverse Curl	10	6-8+	311	or <=10s
EZ on PB				
Incline DB Curl	10	8-10	311	
Horizontal Pull Tri-set:				
Seated Row	10	4-6+	311	tri-set
U/hand grip				i.e. { }
Bent Over Row	10	6-8+	311	or <=10s
(WG/HB)				
Prone DB Fly	10	8-10+	311	
Vertical Pull Tri-set:				
Chin up	10	4-6+	311	tri-set
(palm facing you)				i.e. { }
Lat Pulldown	10	6-8+	311	or <=10s
(WG/B)				
DB Pullover	10	8-10+	311	

Stage 1 : B Day - Exercise Descriptions

Here are descriptions of the exercises involved in B day, Stage 1 of the *Get Buffed!* ™ II (Get More Buffed!) four (4) stage program.

Forearm Flexion : Kneel down in front of a bench, with your wrists supported on the bench, palms up, hands just off the side of the bench. If you are going to use a bilateral movement use a bar, and if you elect to work more unilaterally, use a DB in each hand. In flexion, allow the bar/DB to roll to your fingertips. If you are feeling too much strain on your wrist when using a bar, an EZ bar is a consideration. If the lightest bar in the gym causes you fatigue in the warm up set, it just became the work-set and move on to the next exercise. Use a full range, and terminate the reps if range is lost.

Bicep Tri-set :

Incline DB Curl – Use an incline bench with approximately 45 degree incline for the Incline DB Curls. The elbows should remain behind the body and still throughout. Palms remain supine or facing upwards. Only flex as high as you can without the elbow moving – they should remain behind the body, with the upper arm perpendicular to the ground throughout.

Reverse Curl EZ on PB - Take the EZ bar and sit on the Preacher Bench, using a palm down (prone) medium grip. Place the full length of the upper arm against the preacher bench, with your arm pits into the top of the pad. If the bench is adjustable, use a 45 degree angle. Use a full stretch, but do not come up to a point where the load or tension is reduced.

Seated Hammer DB Curl+Twist - Sit on the end of a prone bench with DBs down by the side, palms facing inwards (neutral grip). As you lift rotate the DBs outwards so that at the top the thumb end of your grip is as externally rotated as it can be without the elbows leaving the side. Reverse this movement during the lower. Lift the DBs up keeping the elbow still and by the side.

Note -

- If you did wanted to do the Reverse curl at least semi-unilaterally, you should use DBs instead of a barbell.
- If you had a serious bilateral imbalance you could choose to do all the above one arm at a time continuously i.e. until all reps completed.

Horizontal Pulling Tri-set :

Prone DB Fly - Lie face down on a bench. Keep the elbows only slightly bent and at a constant angle throughout. Raise the arms up to the side, keeping them approx. 90 degrees to the long axis of the body. Pause at top. Do not rest the hands on the floor between reps, and minimize the upper trap involvement.

Bent Over Row-WG/HB – Stand with your feet shoulder width or slightly wider apart. Bend forward at the waist and push your hips back a bit, so that the center of gravity of your body is as close to directly over the legs as possible. Have the legs slightly bent. Keep the trunk flat in a line or angle slightly above horizontal to the ground, and do not allow this angle to change whatsoever during the lift. Take a wide grip on a barbell and raise it to a high point on your chest. If you are not able to keep your lower arm and wrist in a straight line, pull the bar to a point lower on the body, and/or lower the load being used. Use a full stretch, and ensure you make it to the trunk. Focus on pulling with the shoulder blades, and squeezing them together at the top. If you were preferring a more unilateral movement, you can do this in the same body position using DBs or lying face down on a bench, using DBs.

Seated Row-Underhand (U/H) grip - Using a shoulder width, underhand grip (palm facing up) grip, pulling to the middle of the trunk. If during this movement you feel any upper trap involvement (e.g. shoulders lifting), lower the point on the body you are pulling the bar in towards. Ensure full retraction (pulling together) of shoulder blades at top of movement.

Vertical Pulling Tri-set :

DB Pullover - If you want to exploit a unilateral movement, have one DB in each hand, either lying along bench or across bench on your back. Start with a slight elbow bend and maintain this throughout. Look to have the lats do the work, not the triceps, which will require a focus on the movement coming from the shoulders. How far you lower the DBs depends upon your comfortable range. Most importantly be consistent in your range. Pause and then lift back up to the top, but stop before the arms reach a perpendicular position to the ground. Ensure the arms stay at the same height throughout but do not allow them to touch. If you prefer a bilateral movement do the same with a bar.

Lat Pulldown-WG/B - Take a wide grip on the lat pulldown bar, and pull behind the head to the base of your neck. Ideally use this full range, but you may have conditions that don't allow. Most importantly, be consistent in the range you use. Ideally, at the bottom position your elbows are directly under your wrists. To achieve this, you may find the need to lower the load CONSIDERABLY and to use a spotter who has the courage to tell you the truth! Allow the arms to go to a full stretch in the top position. There will be some whose shoulder laxity or injury/surgery history suggests they should be going to the front rather than behind the head. In this case, apply the same technical tips.

Chin Up – palm facing you - use a supine grip (palm facing your face), shoulder width. Start in a full stretch position with the feet crossed and tucked up. Ensure the chin goes well over the bar, and that you return to the full stretch position. Keep the body sway under control by focusing on control in the lowering phase.

Stage 1, Option 1 – Hypertrophy / Lower Training Age

C Day

Exercise	Warm up	Work	Speed	Rest
Calf press standing, single or double	15	6-8+ 8-10+ 10-12+ 12-15	311	strip set
Leg Curl (single or double)	10	10+10+10	311	strip set
Leg Curl (single or double)	10	10+10+10	311	strip set
Ski squat (single or double)	nil	5x10-60sec	n/a	½-1m
Single leg squat - back foot on bench	10	10	1.5's	½-1m
Single leg squat	nil	1xmax reps	311	1-2m
Pause squats-HB/NS	10	10	331	1-2m
1 ¼ squats-HB/NS	nil	10	1.3	1-2m
Explosive squats-HB/NS	nil	10	30*	1-2m

Stage 1, Option 2 - Hypertrophy-neural / Intermediate Training Age

C Day

Exercise	Warm up	Work	Speed	Rest
Calf press – standing, single or double	12/10	4-6+ 6-8+ 8-10+ 10-12	311	strip set
Leg Curl (single or double)	10	8+8+8	311	strip set
Leg Curl (single or double)	10	8+8+8	311	strip set
Ski squat (single or double)	nil	5x10-60sec	n/a	1m
Single leg squat – back foot on bench	8	8	1.5's	1m
Single leg squat	nil	1xmax reps	311	2m
Pause squats-HB/NS	8	8	331	2m
1 ¼ squats-HB/NS	nil	8	1.3	2m
Explosive squats-HB/NS	nil	8	20*	2m

Stage 1, Option 3 - Neural/Advanced Training Age

C Day

Exercise	Warm up	Work	Speed	Rest
Pause squats-HB/NS	8	8	331	2m
1 ¼ squats-HB/NS	nil	8	1.3	2m
Explosive squats-HB/NS	nil	8	20*	2m
Single leg squat	nil	1xmax reps	311	2m
Single leg squat – back foot on bench	8	8	1.5's	1m
Ski squat (single or double)	nil	5x10-60sec	n/a	1m
Leg Curl (single or double)	10	8+8+8	311	strip set
Leg Ext (single or double)	10	8+8+8	311	strip set
Calf press – standing, single or double	12/10	4-6+ 6-8+ 8-10+ 10-12	311	strip set

Stage 1 : C Day - Exercise Descriptions

Here are descriptions of the exercises involved in C day, Stage 1 of the *Get Buffed!* ™ II (Get More Buffed!) four (4) stage program.

Calf Multi-set : These are all on the standing calf press. Do one leg at a time if you have a bilateral imbalance, two together if this is not an issue. Remember to minimize the movement at ALL other joints in the body, including the arms and shoulders – make the calf's do the work! And use a full range of movement, including a deep stretch. There is some advantage of having non-slip shoes on here, and you may find it best to have your laces done up fairly tightly. There are four sets in this strip set. When you strip down for the next set, aim to select a weight that will allow you to achieve a number of reps within the recommended rep bracket, but don't get too concerned if you work just outside the rep brackets indicated. If you do more or less, the most important thing is that you note it in your training diary and look to do better next time.

Leg Curl/Extension: You decide whether you do this one single or double leg based on your bilateral balance. No matter which of the three programs you use, I recommend doing hamstrings (leg curls) first in Stage 1. The leg curl should be done in a strip set of three sets. With the leg curl, keep the foot orientation neutral throughout and prevent the pelvis from anteriorly rotating during the lift. With the extension, whatever orientation of the foot you start with keep it i.e. do not change the foot orientation during the lift.

Ski Squats : Place your feet shoulder width apart about 2 feet out from the wall, and lean your back against the wall. Bend your knees to a half squat position. This is position one. After a specified time, lower down to position two, about 2 inches lower. After the specified time, lower another 2 inches down to position three. You should be about thigh parallel by now. Use another 2 lower positions, with position five being about as far as you can bend at the knees. How long is the specified time? Start with somewhere between 10-20 seconds per position, adding 5 seconds per workout. The 5 positions done with no rest between them constitutes a set. Just one set on day one remember. If you are finding this too easy or notice one leg doing more work than the other, do it on one leg at a time. The challenge here (apart from the obvious of having twice as much loading on the leg!) is keeping the hips parallel to the ground, as they would be in the double leg version.

Single Leg Squat – back foot on the bench : Face away from a normal height bench, and place your rear leg up on the bench. You can check your distance by having a relatively vertical shin throughout the movement. Keep your chest and trunk vertical throughout. Lower the body down by bending the knee of the lead leg until the knee of the back leg is almost on the ground. Use bodyweight in the warm up, DBs in the hand in the work set. I recommend the 1 ½'s technique here – go all the way down until the knee is brushing but not resting on the ground – pause – then come up half or maybe only one third of the way – pause, then go back down to the bottom knee-to-carpet brush – pause – then come back up all the way to the top but stop short of full extension. Pause. This is one rep. Have a short rest before doing the other leg and of course, do the weak side first!

Single Leg Squat : I want you to do this one single leg exercise, irrespective of your bilateral leg strength balance. As per my 'Weak Side Rule', do your weaker side first. Very simple concept – stand on one leg and squat as far down as your strength or flexibility (or both!) will tolerate. I am going to throw in three options – from the easiest to the most challenging.

   a. On a very reclined hack squat.
   b. Leaning back on to a Swiss ball with the ball up against a wall (just need to position the ball appropriately).

c. Free standing, maybe with a vertical frame nearby to hold for balance.

Generally speaking, I encourage you to pursue range over reps, but initially use a range that allows you to get at least 8-10 reps.

Explosive Squat : Using my squat technique (described below), use a conventional controlled lowering speed, but a deliberately explosive lift, such that you may go to your toes at the end of the concentric phase. If you are losing control of the hips (e.g. hips are rising faster than the shoulders) out of the bottom position, delay the acceleration until you are through the sticking point or joint angle at which your technique breaks down.

1 and a Quarter Squats : This is the same concept as a one and a half (1 ½ or 1.5s) – just instead of coming out of the movement half way, you only come up a quarter of the way. So go all the way down, pause, come up ¼ of the way, pause, go down to the bottom again, pause, then return to the top. Avoid full extension of the knees, pausing at the top – this is one rep.

Pause Squat : Place the bar as high as is comfortable on the neck, take a narrower than shoulder width stance, and allow only a slight external rotation of the feet. Keep the knees equal distance during the lower and lift, go as deep as your flexibility allows, taking 3 seconds to get there. If your trunk flexion exceeds 45 degrees, don't go any deeper. At the bottom, pause for 3 seconds, keeping the muscles around the hip and knee contracted. Then look to return to the starting position at a normal, non-explosive, controlled pace. Avoid full lock out at the top.

Stage 1, Option 1 – Hypertrophy / Lower Training Age

D Day

Exercise	Warm up	Work	Speed	Rest
Forearm Extension	10	8-10+	311	tri-set
(1 or 2 arm)		10-12+	311	i.e. { }
		12-15	311	or <=10s
Tricep Tri-set :				
Overhead Extens.	10	10-12+	311	tri-set
Lying Tricep Extens.	10	8-10+	311	i.e. { }
Dips or bench dips	10	6-8	311	or <=10s
Vertical Push Tri-set:				
Seated Lateral	10	10-12+	311	tri-set
DB Raise				i.e. { }
Seated Arnold Press	10	8-10+	311	or <=10s
Seated Shoulder	10	6-8	311	
Press –WG/B				
Horizontal Push Tri-set:				
Supine DB Fly	10	10-12+	311	tri-set
Decline DB Press	10	8-10+	311	i.e. { }
Incline Bench Press	10	6-8	311	or <=10s
– WG/HB				

Stage 1, Option 2 - Hypertrophy-neural / Intermediate Training Age

D Day

Exercise	Warm up	Work	Speed	Rest
Forearm Extension	10	6-8+	311	tri-set
(1 or 2 arm)		8-10+	311	i.e. { }
		10-12	311	or <=10s
Tricep Tri-set :				
Overhead Extension	10	8-10+	311	tri-set
Lying Tricep Extens.	10	6-8+	311	i.e. { }
Dips or bench dips	10	4-6	311	or <=10s
Vertical Push Tri-set:				
Seated Lateral DB Raise	10	8-10+	311	tri-set i.e. { }
Seated Arnold Press	10	6-8+	311	or <=10s
Seated Shoulder Press–WG/B	10	4-6	311	
Horizontal Push Tri-set:				
Supine DB Fly	10	8-10+	311	tri-set
Decline DB Press	10	6-8+	311	i.e. { }
Incline Bench Press – WG/HB	10	4-6	311	or <=10s

Stage 1, Option 3 - Neural/Advanced Training Age

D Day

Exercise	Warm up	Work	Speed	Rest
Forearm Extension	10	6-8+	311	tri-set
(1 or 2 arm)		8-10+	311	i.e. { }
		10-12	311	or <=10s
Tricep Tri-set :				
Dips or bench dips	10	4-6+	311	tri-set
Lying Tricep Extens.	10	6-8+	311	i.e. { }
Overhead Extension	10	8-10	311	or <=10s
Vertical Push Tri-set:				
Seated Shoulder	10	4-6+	311	tri-set
Press–WG/B				i.e. { }
Seated Arnold Press	10	6-8+	311	or <=10s
Seated Lateral	10	8-10+	311	
DB Raise				
Horizontal Push Tri-set:				
Incline Bench Press	10	4-6+	311	tri-set
– WG/HB				i.e. { }
Decline DB Press	10	6-8+	311	or <=10s
Supine DB Fly	10	8-10+	311	

Stage 1 : D Day - Exercise Descriptions

Here are descriptions of the exercises involved in D day, Stage 1 of the *Get Buffed!* ™ II (Get More Buffed!) four (4) stage program.

Forearm Extension: Kneel down in front of a bench, with your wrists supported on the bench, palms down, hands just off the side of the bench. If you are going to use a bilateral movement use a bar, and if you elect to work more unilaterally, use a DB in each hand. In extension, ensure you extend as high as the joint will allow without the forearm leaving the bench whatsoever – and be consistent with this range! If you are feeling too much strain on your wrist when using a bar, an EZ bar is a consideration.

Tricep Tri-set :

Overhead Extension – To be done seated, using DBs or a bar. Raise the bar or DB straight over your head, elbow beside the ears. Keep the elbow as high and as far back as possible at all times (to maximize the stretch on the tricep) and keep the elbow to the ear. If using DBs, use a range that results in the DB touching the upper back.

Lying Tricep Extension – Lie on your back on the bench. Raise the bar over your head, arms out stretched. Start with the upper arm slightly behind the vertical, and the head slightly off the end of the bench. Do not let the elbow or upper arm position change from there during the movement. Lower the bar to the top of the forehead. You can use a bar or DBs.

Dips or Bench Dip - If your triceps are not up to it, do bench dips (between 2 benches). Otherwise, use a medium width (just outside shoulders) parallel bar. Cross the feet at the ankles, bend the knees so the ankles are at or near knee height. Lower down until the shoulders are lower than the elbow joint (providing you have no joint or injury conditions that contraindicate this). Keep the body still during the lift and lower, so the movement is not affected by momentum. Do not lock out fully at the top.

Note -
- If you wanted to do the Overhead extension or the Lying Tricep Extension at least semi-unilaterally, you should use DBs instead of a barbell.
- If you had a serious bilateral imbalance you could chose to do all the above one arm at a time continuously i.e. until all reps completed.

Vertical Pushing Tri-set :

Seated Lateral DB Raise - Sit at the end of a bench with the feet together. Hold DBs by the side. With a slightly bent elbow, raise the arms and DBs up to the side keeping the little finger just a little higher than the thumb. Stop at about top of head height, and then lower back down.

Arnold DB Shoulder Press - Sit on a bench with feet apart forming a triangle with your hips. Hold DBs in each hand at shoulder level. In the bottom position, the DBs will be facing your ears. As you lift to full or near-full extension of the arms, slowly rotate the DBs out until they are facing out as much as you can rotate them in the top position. Reverse this during the lowering.

Seated Shoulder Press – WG/B – Take a barbell from the squat rack as you would a squat (on your shoulders) and sit on a bench with feet apart forming a triangle with your hips. With a wide grip on the bar, press the bar up evenly but avoid full lock out. When you lower down, do so to a consistent point on the back of the neck, preferably to the base of the neck. As with the Lat Pulldown to the back of the neck, there may be some whose shoulder condition limits their range or precludes them from this lift. Be sensible. During the lift keep the bar in line – losing line in this lift can be stressful on the neck. When I say in line, I mean in a consistent line of movement. Deviating from this line is 'getting out of line'.

Horizontal Pushing Tri-set :

Supine DB Fly - Lie on your back on a bench, DB in each hand. Hold the DBs directly above your chest, with elbows slightly bent. As you lower and lift this elbow angle is not to change. Lower to as full a range as is comfortable and safe, and most importantly, be consistent with the range. When it comes to range you may have decide where your priorities are – with range or load. In the early stages you may not be able to have both, and I recommend range. Return the DBs to the start position, keeping in mind the option of not bringing them up fully. This will keep the tension on the muscle, and increase the degree of fatigue.

Decline DB Press - Place the decline at a low angle (again about 30 degrees). Hold the DBs with the thumbs facing in, and make sure you use a full stretch. Lower to as big a stretch as you can get, and press the DBs towards each other at the top. Avoid full lockout, and use a spotter when going near fatigue.

Incline Bench Press – WG/HB – Using an incline bench angle of about 30 degrees, take a wide grip on the bar. Lower the bar to a position high on the chest (i.e. high on the sternum). When you press back up, avoid full lockout. Again, get a spotter when using loads likely to cause high level fatigue.

Stage 1 – Concluding Comments

Stage 1 of the program may come across complex, but I do encourage you to study it closely before you do it. Rushing into it will guarantee in a misinterpretation. Study it right down to the finer technical issues. I will leave you with two pearls of wisdom : firstly, if in doubt – do less! And secondly and finally, having a four (4) stage plan prepared in advance will almost always give you better results than making it up as you go!

As far as your tailoring this program to suit your individual needs, use the guidelines that I provide earlier in this book. Yes, there were more complexities in deciding which program to use and how to put it together than you have experienced in getting programs for your usual 'muscle and fiction' magazines – but then the results are going to be different – significantly better! And you can take a lot of credit for that because you put the effort in to interpret the options; you analyzed your body and your training history; you had the courage to do something different than what you have done in the past and very different to what the 'majority' are doing. And you were the one that is going to get the results!

Stage 2

Stage 2 – Overview

Again in Stage 2 the lower body dominates over the upper body if you use linear periodization. If you are using the alternating approach the upper body will be dominating.

So what's in store in Stage 2?

The **abdominal program** in this stage is placed first in the workout. If you are lacking in the abdominal strength and control, I would recommend you retain this sequence. In Stages 3 and 4, provided you have achieved your minimal abdominal standards, you could move them to the back of the workout. But you can and should be making this decision as you go based on the progress and standard you expect in your abdominal strength and control.

In the **lower body program** in this stage the hip dominance is continued, by placing the hip movements earlier in the week than the quad dominant movements. However the sequence of exercises within the workout is more conventional, going from bigger muscle group, more loaded exercises to smaller muscle group, less loaded movements.

In the **upper body program** in this stage we go back to pushing and pulling in the one workout. You will also be working vertical pushing and pulling early in the training week and horizontal pushing and pulling later. This means that the vertical work is prioritized in this phase – which is unusual because most people most of the time will prioritize horizontal work in general, horizontal pushing in particular.

I have continued to give priority to what I have observed is most strength training participants greatest weaknesses – their pulling muscles, or more specifically their ability to pull in horizontal (scapula retract) and vertical (scapula depress) planes.

On the horizontal push-pull day, horizontal pulling dominates (by appearing earlier in the sequence) over horizontal pushing. Another hard pill to swallow for those connected by their umbilical cords to benching first in the workout! Trust me, a short-term de-emphasizing of benching will create a long-term boost!

You will also note that upper arms are no longer prioritized over the core pushing/pulling muscles as they were in stage one. Hopefully, the increased size and strength gained from prioritizing the elbow flexors/extensors in the earlier stage will boost strength capacity in this and subsequent stages – this is the goal.

Most of the upper body program in this stage is based on **alternate setting**. The way I want you to do this is do a set of one exercise, rest as long as you feel you need to, and then do a set of the next exercise, rest again for as long as you need to, then repeat this cycle. So you will complete all the sets for 2 exercises before moving on. How long is 'rest long enough'? A general guideline for work sets (warm up sets require less) might be :

- Hypertrophy/Lower training age option : 1-2 minutes.
- Hypertrophy-neural/Intermediate Training Age Option : 2-3 minutes.
- Neural/Advanced Training Age Option : 3-4 minutes.

There are some exercises where you will just take a **normal standard set/rest** approach, usually the last exercise in a program that has an odd number of exercises e.g. the Neural/Advanced Training Age Option.

When you get the **strip sets** in some of the exercises, look to use 3 different loads (heavy to light) and conclude the set in the number of reps indicated. For example if it asks for 12-15, you may do 4-6 on each of 3 different loads. If your load selection turns out to be at the upper end of your capability, which I would expect in week 3 of this stage, use the 10 sec rest period available. If your load selection turns out to be at the lower end of your capability, which I would expect in week 1 of this stage, use little or no rest between the 3 different loads.

The following provides **general information about this stage of the program**:

Note that the 6/1/6/1 or 5/1/5/1 loading model is used in this phase. Both are based on the same concept – the aim of the first 1 x 6 (or 1 x 5) is to enhance the loading potential of second 1 x 6 (or 1 x 5). The aim of the first 1 x 1 is also aimed at raising the loading potential of the second 1 x 6 (or 1 x 5), as well as the loading potential of the second 1 x 1. So the second 1 x 6 (or 1 x 5) and 1 x 1 are aimed at exploiting the neural dis-inhibition created by the first 1 x 6 (or 1x5) and 1 x 1. If you don't respect this – that is, if you go too heavy in the first 1 x 6 (or 1x 5) and or 1 x 1, you will not experience this neural dis-inhibition, as it will be clouded by fatigue. Here is an example of what I recommend :

Sample loading pattern in week 1 for the 6/1/6/1 method:

1 x 6 @ 100 kg

1 x 1 @ 125 kg

1 x 6 @ 105 kg

1 x 1 @ 130 kg

Then in the next week, the second 6 (or 5) and 1 become the first set loading – see below:

Sample loading pattern in week 2 for the 6/1/6/1 method:

1 x 6 @ 105 kg

1 x 1 @ 130 kg

1 x 6 @ 110 kg

1 x 1 @ 135 kg

Of course, if there is a third week, the same technique applies but the increments don't need to be as high. For example:

Sample loading pattern in week 3 for the 6/1/6/1 method:

1 x 6 @ 110 kg

1 x 1 @ 135 kg

1 x 6 @ 112.5 kg

1 x 1 @ 137.5 kg

Now go and *Get Buffed!*™

Stage 2 – Warm Up / Stretching / Abdominal / Control Drills

A & C Day

Exercise	Warm up	Work	Speed	Rest
Warm Up	10-20 minutes of light aerobic type activity e.g. stationary bike			
Stretch	20-40 minutes of lower body stretching			
Abdominals				
Knee up on flat or incline	nil	1-2x10-20	311 or 5 sec holds	30-60s
Knees to sky	nil	1-2x10	5sec hold	30-60s
Side raises on Roman Chair	nil	1-2x10-15 per side	311	30-60s
Seated thin tummy / / squeeze cheeks and lift alternate leg	nil	1-2x10-15 lifts per leg	leg lift-202	30-60s
Control Drills				
Light leg extensions	nil	1x15-20	202	0-30s
Prone lying single leg hip / thigh extensions	nil	1x15-25	202	0-30s
Side Lying Lateral Leg Raise	nil	1x15-25	202	0-30s
Co-Contraction Lunge	nil	1x10-20	202	0-30s
Lying Supine Single Leg Hip/Thigh Extension	nil	1x5-15	202	0-30s
Assisted Squat	nil	1x10	202	0-30s

Workout

Stage 2 : A & C Day – Abdominal Exercise Descriptions

Here are descriptions of the abdominal exercises involved in A and C day, Stage 2 of the *Get Buffed!* ™ II (Get More Buffed!) four (4) stage program.

Knee Up on flat or incline : In this exercise you get to choose between the lower level of difficulty of lying on the ground, or the higher level of difficulty of lying on an incline abdominal bench or similar. If you chose the incline bench, you have another decision to make as to what angle to set the incline at.

Lie on your back on the ground or on the incline abdominal bench. Bring your knees and hips to 90 degrees of flexion. Now press you lower back flat against the floor or bench (ideally using your 'lower abdominals'). Now lift your knees to your chest, maintaining the 90 degree knee angle. Once there lower the legs down allowing them to extend as soon as you start lowering. Lower down until your legs are almost parallel to the ground or bench. Do not rest the legs on the floor or bench between reps.

So how do you decide which surface to use? Comes down to your perception of quality. If you wanted to apply a higher standard, you would only use a surface or incline that would allow you to maintain a posteriorly rotated pelvis (top of pelvis pulled backwards) all the way during the lowering. Bottom line is there is a difference between what you can do and what you can do well, and in the absence of supervision I am realistic as to what the outcomes may be.

I also know that the incline abdominal boards are not as prevalent in gyms now as perhaps previously. You may need to improvise. One simple way is to place one end of a prone bench on a low block, or to gain adjustable options, on a Reebok step. Lie on the bench with you head at the higher end, holding the bench either side of your ears with your hands.

Notes :

Speed of movement – Controlled dynamic movement at 313.

Selecting appropriate level – Trial and error. In this exercise you really need to educate yourself to feel for when they lose the 'set' position of the pelvis.

Knees to Sky : This is a more advanced version of the toes to sky from the prior stage. If you feel you have not mastered the prior version, perhaps continue on with it. Remember this movement is not as 'fine' in its requirements as the above in relation to making the tummy thin.

Lie on your back, arms out on the ground at 90 degrees to the trunk, have your legs together, and bend your knees and hips to 90 degrees of flexion, so that your upper legs are vertical and your lower legs are parallel to the ground.

I identify at least three levels of difficulty in this drill. Ideally you would have mastered Level 1 and or 2 in the first Stage, and be focusing on Level 3 in this program, Stage 2.

Level 1 - lift the pelvis as far off the ground whilst maintaining totally vertical leg   position (initially this may not be very far at all, at even at best the   movement is limited in its range) and hold for 5-10 seconds.

Level 2 - as above, but bend one knee to 90 degrees at knee; alternate each rep which leg is bent, which is straight.

Level 3 - as above, but bend both knees so that the knees are bent to 90 degrees.

Notes :

Speed of movement – A controlled lift, a steady hold for 5-10 seconds; no use of momentum, keeping legs (or upper leg at least) always totally vertical.

Arm positions - Keep arms out to side on ground, 90 degrees to trunk.

Selecting appropriate level – Trial and error.

Side Raises on Roman Chair : This is a slightly different body position, but a progression from and offers a higher level of difficulty than the previous lateral trunk flexion exercise on the ground as used in Stage 1.

Lie on your side on a bench or a device known as the Roman Chair. The bench or Roman Chair supports your hips and legs, and your trunk is off the bench. In the case of a normal bench, you will need someone to hold your feet. In the case of the Roman Chair, hook your feet under the heel pad. Lower the body down, maintaining this sideways position. Go as far down as is safe and comfortable, and return to the starting position. The placement of the hands will alter the level of difficulty. The further the hands are above the head, the harder the movement. In the initial position, have the athlete cross the arms across the chest. Placement of external resistance (e.g. weight plate, med ball etc) on chest is another method for increasing loading.

Notes :

Speed of movement – A controlled lift, say a speed of 311 or 211.

Arm positions - Start with arms crossed on chest but take out further above head as is needed to provide appropriate loading.

Selecting appropriate level – Trial and error.

Seated Thin Tummy/Squeeze Cheeks and lift alternate leg :
Sit on the end of a prone bench, or even on a Swiss ball (there you go – shows I don't dislike them to the point of exclusion!) with your knees and feet together, feet on the ground, chest up and back straight. Now create that thin dish abdominal position I described in the thin tummy drill (Stage 1) – make the lower abdominals thin and contract the lower abdominals. Place your fingers on your tummy just under the belt line, each hand angling in at 45 degrees, with about 4 inches between the fingers on each hand. Use your hands for feedback on the quality of this contraction. Now also squeeze your cheeks in a manner that results in you 'levitating' a inch or so off the bench! You may find that sucking up the pelvic floor contributes to the quality of the contraction!

With that foundation, raise one leg off the ground a few inches in a controlled manner before lowering it down. During this action, maintain the abdominals and cheek tension, the thinness of the abdominals, and the parallel, flat line between the two hips. Then do the other leg in the same way.

Notes :

Speed of movement – Set the abs and cheeks and then conduct 10-15 lifts per leg in a continual manner.

Arm positions – In your abdominal region, getting feedback (same as for thin tummy drill).

Selecting appropriate level – Just the one! If you found this too easy, you could do the same thing standing with your upper back on the bench or ball, and your trunk parallel to the ground. If you struggle with the quality of the movement, do less reps at a higher quality.

Stage 2 – Warm Up / Stretching / Abdominal / Control Drills

B & D Day

Exercise	Warm up	Work	Speed	Rest
Warm Up	optional 5-15 minutes of light aerobic type activity e.g. stationary bike			
Stretch	10-20 minutes of upper body stretching			
Abdominals				
Curl up for rhythm	nil	1-2x15-30	311	30-60s
Bar Roll outs	nil	1-2x10-20	311	30-60s
Russian twist	nil	1-2x15-30 full rotations	202	30-60s
Push up position on Hands -Alternate arm/leg lifts	nil	1x5-15	5s holds	0-30s
Control Drills				
Flutters	nil	1x10-20	202	0-30s
Scarecrow	nil	1x 5-15	202	0-30s
Side Lying Ext DB Rotation	nil	1x10-20	202	0-30s
Prone Limited Range DB Row	nil	1x10-20	202	0-30s

Workout

Stage 2 : B & D Day – Abdominal Exercise Descriptions

Here are descriptions of the abdominal exercises involved in B and D day, Stage 2 of the *Get Buffed!* ™ II (Get More Buffed!) four (4) stage program.

Curl Up for rhythm : Lie on your back on the ground, knees bent to about 90 degrees, and feet flat on the floor. Your feet are not to be anchored under anything. Then you sit up or curl up the trunk, ideally to a full sitting position.

In this stage I want you to do sit-ups for numbers i.e. looking to increase work capacity, but not allowing total fatigue or excessive slowing of movement. If the consistent speed of movement drops, terminate.

Notes :

Speed of movement – I like to see a rigid adherence to pre-determined speed in this phase e.g. 3 down, 1 pause, 1 up.

Arm positions - Each of these levels of difficulty have at least 5 different arm positions that provide further variety/levels of difficulty
> 1 = arms remain parallel to ground, pointed towards feet
> 2 = upper arms remain parallel to ground, hands on opposite elbow
> 3 = upper arms remain parallel to ground, hands on opposite shoulder
> 4 = hands touching forehead, elbows out at 45 degrees to front of head
> 5 = hands touching side of head, elbows forming a straight line either side

Selecting appropriate level – Trial and error.

Bar Roll Outs : Kneel on the ground, placing a barbell with at least small plates (2.5-5 kgs) on each end on the ground in front of you. Grip the barbell with your hands shoulder width. Keeping your arms relatively straight, roll the bar out in front of you and lower your trunk down towards the ground. If you can, go all the way down till your body is nearly touching but not resting on the ground. (what I mean is if you can come up from there – going down is the easy part!). Only use the downward range you can recover upwards from!

The key technical point is that as you lower and more particularly as you lift, keep the hips and trunk in line. That is, your body should form a straight line between your knees and shoulders at all times. Resist the temptation to stick your hips in the air, particularly during the up phase. Yes, there will be a degree of arm and upper trunk strength/work involved!

Notes :

Speed of movement – Control down in about 2-3 seconds, lift as fast as you can without losing the appropriate line between the knee and hip.

Arm positions – Keep the arms relatively straight and do not change the elbow angle during the movement.

Selecting appropriate level – The variable you control is mainly how far you go down. Only go down (trunk towards the ground) as far as you can come up from in the manner recommended. Another variable may be the height of the bar off the ground, but I suggest using only 2.5 kg – 5 kg plates.

Russian Twist : Lie on your back on the ground or in a suitable device. Have your knees bent to 90 degrees, feet flat. Feet can be anchored (hooked under) or not. Lean the trunk back to a 45 degree angle or further. Keep the spine as straight as possible. Rotate the trunk from side to side along this axis. Where greater resistance is desired, hold a medicine ball or weight plate out at 90 degrees from the angle of the trunk. The further the load is held from the body the greater the resistance.

Notes :

Speed of movement – A controlled lift, say a speed of 303 or 202

Arm positions - The position of the hands will influence the load. The easiest load will be with the arm crossed on the chest. The further the load is held from the body the greater the resistance.

Selecting appropriate level – Use trial and error. Do not continue on looking for failure – work with a level that is manageable. For example, do not allow arms to bend, to change angle relative to body, to round the back, or to rotate only from the arms instead of the waist.

Push Up Position on Hands - alternate arm/leg lifts : Go face down on the ground on your hands and feet in a push up position. A rep will be each time you lift a leg or arm. When you lift the leg or arm (or in some cases both), lift only till they are in line with the trunk, and aim to keep the trunk flat throughout the lift. You can manipulate the difficulty of this exercise by which variation or level you select from below. Count each time you lift a limb as a rep. You can also vary the duration that the limb/s is/are held up.

Notes :

Speed of movement – Hold each limb raise for five seconds. Recover for 1-2 seconds at the bottom position (resting in push up position between reps).

Arm positions - Start with the arms under the shoulders, shoulder width. Levels of difficulty for alternate limb lifting include :

1 = Raise one arm only, then the other only, then one leg only, then the other only etc.

2 = Raise opposite arm and leg simultaneously.

3 = Raise opposite arm and leg simultaneously and abduct in the plane that the body is in for 45 degrees (legs) and 90 degrees (arms).

Selecting appropriate level – When you fall flat on your face you know you have gone too far! Seriously, before that occurs you will be changing the shape of the body (varying from the recommended parallel to ground through the body position) and this is not what I am looking for.

Stage 2, Option 1 - Hypertrophy / Lower Training Age

A Day

Exercise	Warm up	Work	Speed	Rest
Deadlift (MG/O-hand)	1x10 / 1x8	6/1/6/1	311	3-4m
Deadlift (MG/SOB)	nil or 1x4	1x12-15	311	2-3m
Stiff Legged D/lift (WG/Chest up/Flat back)	1x10	1x10	311	2m
King Deadlift (Bent knee/ single leg)	nil	1xamrap	311	2m
Shrug (MG/O-hand)	1x10	1-2x8-10	311	1-2m

Stage 2, Option 2 - Hypertrophy-neural / Intermediate Training Age

A Day

Exercise	Warm up	Work	Speed	Rest
Deadlift (MG/O-hand)	1x10 / 1x8	5/1/5/1	311	3-4m
Deadlift (MG/SOB)	nil or 1x4	1x10-12	311	2-3m
Stiff Legged D/lift (WG/Chest up/Flat back)	1x8	1x8	311	2m
King Deadlift (single leg/bent knee)	nil	1xamrap	311	2m
Shrug (MG/O-hand)	1x8	1-2x6-8	311	1-2m

Stage 2, Option 3 - Neural/Advanced Training Age

A Day

Exercise	Warm up	Work	Speed	Rest
Deadlift (MG/O-hand)	1x10 / 1x8	5/1/5/1	311	4m
Deadlift (MG/SOB)	nil or 1x4	1x8-10	311	3-4m
Stiff Legged D/lift (WG/Chest up/flat back)	1x6	1x6	311	3m
King Deadlift (single leg/bent knee)	nil	1xamrap	311	2-3m
Shrug (MG/O-hand)	1x6	1-2x5-6	311	2m

Stage 2 : A Day - Exercise Descriptions

Here are descriptions of the exercises involved in A day, Stage 2 of the *Get Buffed!* ™ II (Get More Buffed!) four (4) stage program.

Deadlifts – MG : Use a medium (just outside your legs), palm over grip, and starting from the bottom position, weight rested on the ground. Now that you are starting to lift more load in this exercise, it is critical you confirm your technique :

Start Position :

1. Feet shoulder width apart.
2. Bar on shins.
3. Shoulders vertically over the bar.
4. Back flat, pelvis and head aligned with spine.
5. Scapula retracted and depressed.

Get Set : (immediately prior to take-off)

1. Extend legs slightly to take up slack (tension on the bar).
2. Suck tummy thin (ensuring pelvis neutral with spine, not arched or rounded).
3. Squeeze cheeks (to assist in above, and add focus to the point that this is where I want the drive to come from).
4. Raise tension in upper back, where scapula position is to be held.

Take off : (first pull = from ground to just above knees)

1. Extend the legs, imaging pushing legs through the ground using gluts as prime mover.
2. As legs extend, trunk angle does not change (stays at same angle as in start) i.e. hips do not raise faster than shoulders - evenly slightly!).
3. Upper back maintained in a flat position (scapula retracted/depressed).
4. Bar stays in contact with skin at all times.

5. Drive with legs - back is a stabilizer!

Second Pull :(from just above knees to standing)

1. Now you stand up, forcing hips through with drive from gluteals.
2. Bar stays in contact with skin at all times.
3. Finish in upright position (no need to hyperextend trunk or roll shoulders!).
4. If upper back position held throughout, shoulders will be down and back in finish position automatically.

Lowering :

1. Unlike most exercises (including the squat) the eccentric phase of the deadlift is not a mirror reverse of the concentric phase.
2. As a general comment, unless I see the specific need, I do not place as much importance on the lowering of the deadlift as I would in other lifts, such as the squat.

Focus on using the gluts out of the bottom position. If you are experiencing lower back pain or excessive fatigue, you are using a technique different to what I recommend - I want all the work in the gluts and the legs. The back is mainly a stabilizer.

Remember, the deadlift provides an unequaled opportunity to balance the upper back in the horizontal plane (pulling) with the front of the upper trunk (chest, or horizontal pushing). Don't miss out on this opportunity – focus on holding the shoulder blades together during the lift (scapula retraction)!

Some of you may also want to revert at this stage to an alternated grip (one hand over, one hand under). This grip really does need to be mastered by those planning to ultimately go heavy in this lift later in this program, and by those hoping to compete in powerlifting. If you are or plan to compete in Olympic weightlifting, using straps in a symmetrical overhand grip may be a more specific option, but no one should rush to use the straps until they can no longer grip the bar i.e. the bar is sliding out of their hands. To assist in gripping the bar I strongly recommend using chalk on your palms also.

Now if you are deadlifting in the way I want (in contact with the skin all the way up), you may experience some skin damage and perhaps even bleed as a result of this. Keep doing this! That is keep the bar close to the body! To reduce the skin damage, consider the following:

- There is such a thing as too rough a bar. You want a bar with enough knurling to support the grip (inadequately knurled bars will slide out of your hands real quick!) but no so rough that you could use it to sand back timber! These extremely rough bars are not overly common but they do exist.
- Wear track pants. This will provide some protection from the bar on the skin. Yes, may mean a warmer workout (but on the other side it keeps the knee and hips warm), and yes, it does mean you cannot get the same crowd effect when you 'accidentally' flex the quads at the water fountain....

If you are not using full size rubber plates (or rubber bumpers), which bring the bar to mid-shin on the average height adult, I want you to place blocks or similar under the plates to create a similar starting height. Let's say you are only using the standard 10kg steel plates on each end, which are approximately half the height of a 20 kg plate. If these steel plates were to be resting on the ground, you would have a very low starting position. It is unlikely (unless you have superior hip flexibility) that you would be able to set the body in the start position that I ask for when required to start from such a low position. If this is the case, place blocks or similar under the bar until the bar is at the height if would be if you had the standard 20 kg rubber plates on. To check this, stand a 20 kg rubber plate, bumper or even a steel plate (provided it is full height) up against the bar when it is on the blocks to confirm it is the same height i.e. the bar is aligned with the hole in the middle of the 20 kg plate.

Deadlifts – MG/SOB : This is as per above but by virtue of the small 'adjustment' (which I am about to explain) and the higher reps, prepare to go back a far way in load on the bar.

This deadlift variation requires you to stand on a block, with the weight position unchanged, resting on the floor. How high the block is that you are to stand on is dependant on your flexibility and ability to create what I would call an appropriate starting position. For most, this means you would stand on a 20 kg full size plate, and even for some, this may be too much for their flexibility and ability to set in the start. However, most will be okay standing on a 1 x 20 kg plate, and the more advanced technically or flexibility wise, may be able to stand on 2 x 20 kilo plates.

Stiff Legged Deadlift – WG/chest up : In this version, the movement starts from the top, in a standing position. Hold the bar with a wide grip (grip outside the line markings on an Olympic type bar), bend the knees slightly, but don't allow the knee angle to change during the lift. Now as you flex forward at the waist, keep the chest up, push the bum backwards, and allow your weight to drift to the heels of your feet. As you go down maintain this flat back position, or even slightly arched in the lower back. Now, if you want to totally isolate the hamstrings in this lift, only go down as far as you can with the hips and spine staying aligned. When you reach the end of your hamstring flexibility or ability to anteriorly rotate the pelvis (i.e. pushing the top of the pelvis forward and the lower end of the pelvis backwards), you will probably still be able to flex the trunk forward by bending at the base of spine – don't! Leave the range at that. As you return to the standing position, consciously contract your gluts and push through with the hips to finish. This technique aims to increase the isolation of the hamstrings. It has not about safety!

King Deadlift : This is a single leg bent knee deadlift. Stand on one leg (starting with the weak side) and bend the other leg up until the lower leg is parallel to the ground. Hands on hips or by side. The aim is to bend the knee of the supporting leg until the knee of the non-supporting leg is brushing the ground. In reality, you may have to settle for a shorter range (you'll understand why I say this as soon as you do this workout). If this is the case - and I expect it will be - look to increase the range from workout to workout.

You are allowed to flex (bend) forward at the waist as much as you want, and doing so will increase the gluteal involvement. Keep the working knee aligned neutrally throughout the movement. Take 3 seconds to lower, 1 second pause each end and 2 seconds to lift. No warm up set needed. When you can do more than 15-20 reps FULL RANGE look to hold DBs in the hands.

Shrug – MG : In a standing position holding a bar in front of the body, take an overhand medium grip (just outside the body). As you shrug the bar upwards with your upper traps, avoid any bending at the elbow or extension of the head. To help with the elbow, turn the elbow joint to face outwards and then consciously push the inside of the elbow joint inwards (using the triceps). To assist the head position, keep the chin in, the head neutral, and chest up. I want to see a flat back horizontally across the shoulder blades in the top position, not a round upper back. You can use wrist straps if you feel you need to, but only if you are no longer able to grip the bar for the duration of the set.

Stage 2, Option 1 – Hypertrophy / Lower Training Age

B Day

Exercise	Warm up	Work	Speed	Rest
Shoulder Press (WG/B)	10/8	6/1/6/1	311	alternate with chin up
Chin Up (WG/overhand)	10/8	6/1/6/1	311	alternate with s/press
Seated Lat DB Raise	opt 1x10	1x6-8+ 1x6-8+ 1x6-8	311	strip set alternate with bi curl
Standing EZ bar Reverse Bi Curl	1x10	1-2x8-10	311	alternate with lat raise

Stage 2, Option 2 - Hypertrophy-neural / Intermediate Training Age

B Day

Exercise	Warm up	Work	Speed	Rest
Shoulder Press (WG/B)	10/8	5/1/5/1	311	alternate with chin up
Chin Up (WG/overhand)	10/8	5/1/5/1	311	alternate with s/press
Seated Lat DB Raise	opt 1x10	1x12-15	311	alternate with bi curl
Standing EZ bar Reverse Bi Curl	1x10	1-2x6-8	311	alternate with lat raise

Stage 2, Option 3 - Neural/Advanced Training Age

B Day

Exercise	Warm up	Work	Speed	Rest
Shoulder Press (WG/B)	10/8/6	4/1/4/1 1x10-15	311	alternate with chin up
Chin Up (WG/overhand)	10/8	4/1/4/1 1x10-15	311	alternate with s/press
Dips	1x10 b/dips	1-2x5-6 Opt 1x10	311	2-3mins

Stage 2 : B Day - Exercise Descriptions

Here are descriptions of the exercises involved in B day, Stage 2 of the *Get Buffed!* ™ II (Get More Buffed!) four (4) stage program.

Seated Shoulder Press – *WG/B* : Take a barbell from the squat racks and sit on a bench with feet apart forming a triangle with your bum. With a wide grip on the bar, press the bar up evenly but avoid full lock out. When you lower down, do so to a consistent point on the back of the neck, preferably to the base of the neck. As with the Lat Pulldown to the back of the neck, there may be some whose shoulder condition limits their range or precludes them from this lift. Be sensible. During the lift keep the bar in line – losing line in this lift can be stressful on the neck. When I say in line, I mean in a consistent line of movement. Deviating from this line is 'getting out of line'.

The hardest part about starting a shoulder press is getting it off the shoulders for the first rep. Which is why I suspect so many chose to start the movement from the top. I may be a bit old-fashioned, but I like to also develop the strength to start from a dead-stop off the bottom. Which is why I usually do them this way.

This challenge of getting the bar going really increases the need for and benefit of learning how to 'hold your breath' and keep the torso 'up and tight'. If you attempt to start the rep off with a body like a rag doll, you will display the strength of one!

Note that with using a wide grip, as the load increases there may be a tendency for the hands to slip out along the bar. Negate this with the use of chalk.

Remember also that the shoulder press, relative to other bigger muscle lifts, deals in smaller numbers. So a 2.5 kg increase may represent a large percentage increase in load. Respect this and use appropriate increments. Do your sums to help, and don't be down on yourself for achieving only small increments week to week in this lift. 'Even the little fish are sweet!'

Chin Up – prone/WG : Use a prone grip (palm facing away), shoulder width. Start in a full stretch position with the feet crossed and tucked up. Ensure the chin goes well over the bar, and that you return to the full stretch position keeping the body sway under control. What constitutes a wide grip? A medium grip for me is the hand space just outside the shoulder. A wide grip is the next hand space out from that.

Note that many gyms have the chin bars that drop off diagonally towards the ground at the ends. Whilst I suspect this may be more ergonomically correct, I don't like or recommend them. Two things. The hand grips at this area are usually too wide for the average person, and secondly, you are not likely to have the horizontal bar section as a guide to maintain consistent range in the concentric phase. I am happy for you to use a straight chin bar, or the horizontal part of the chin bar if it does drop off.

The loading protocol in this phase is going to require the use of external loading. There are many ways of doing this, and I am going to share with you my preferred method. I simply get a meter of rope, tie a reef knot connecting each end. Then I insert the first end of the loop through the center of a weight plate, and the second end of the loop through the first end of the loop. Then through the second end of the loop I insert the tongue of a 4" weight belt. Ideally the rope is short enough so that the weight plate is hanging just below the crotch. I then clamp the weight plate between my thighs. May sound like a lot of mucking around but the main thing is to get the weight plate in line with my center of gravity and not swaying about at all. You may be surprised at the positive difference this or similar positioning may have on your chins!

Should you use wrist straps to anchor your hands to the chin bar? I would suggest not at this phase. Again I may be old fashioned but I like the added benefit of the training effect of gripping on the forearm strength and size!

Seated Lateral DB Raise : Sit at the end of a bench with the feet together. Hold DBs by the side. With a slightly bent elbow, raise the arms and DBs up to the side keeping the little finger just a little higher than the thumb. Stop at about top of head height, and then lower back down.

As the loads increase into this phase there may be the temptation to cheat a bit more on this set – do your best to resist this temptation! But if it happens on the last rep or so of the set, so be it.

Standing EZ Reverse Bicep Curl : Grab the EZ bar with a palm down (prone) medium (shoulder width) grip. Slightly bend or more accurately unlock the knees and keep them there. This will reduce the ability to extend through the trunk, increasing arm isolation. Starting with the arms fully extended and keeping the arms by the side, bend (flex) the elbows until the bar is just before the 'gravity line'. This is the point at which you might feel significant downturn in resistance. Going into this area increases the rest period, which is not bad, but from a bodybuilding perspective I believe you stay just short of this point. Then lower the bar back down to the fully extended elbow position.

There may be a temptation to avoid full extension, and there may be times when this technique is appropriate from a hypertrophy perspective. However from an injury prevention perspective I would encourage predominantly the use of full extension in elbow flexion exercises. The concern is potential shortening of the elbow flexors.

As per the seated Lateral DB Raise look to resist the temptation to cheat, but if it happens on the last rep or 2 in a slight way, no serious implications!

Note in the Neural/Advanced Training Age Option for the second upper body program in the week, this exercise is performed at the end of D day.

Stage 2, Option 1 – Hypertrophy / Lower Training Age

C Day

Exercise	Warm up	Work	Speed	Rest
Squat (MB/MS)	1x10/1x8	6/1/6/1	301	2-3m
Squat (NS/HB)	nil	1x12-15	1.5's	2-3m
Dynamic Lunge (bar on back)	1x10/leg	1x10/leg	10*	2m
Single leg squat	nil	1xAMRAP	311	2m
Calf press (standing/double leg)	1x15	1-2x12-15	311	1-2m

Stage 2, Option 2 - Hypertrophy-neural / Intermediate Training Age

C Day

Exercise	Warm up	Work	Speed	Rest
Squat (MB/MS)	1x10/1x8	5/1/5/1	301	3-4m
Squat (NS/HB)	nil	1x10-12	1.5's	3m
Dynamic Lunge (-bar on back)	1x8/leg	1x8/leg	10*	2-3m
Single leg squat	nil	1xAMRAP	311	2m
Calf press (standing/double leg)	1x12	1-2x10-12	311	1-2m

Stage 2, Option 3 - Neural/Advanced Training Age

C Day

Exercise	Warm up	Work	Speed	Rest
Squat (MB/MS)	1x10/1x8	5/1/5/1	301	4m
Squat (NS/HB)	nil	1x8-10	1.5's	3-4m
Dynamic Lunge (bar on back)	1x6/leg	1x6/leg	10*	3m
Single leg squat	nil	1xAMRAP	311	2-3m
Calf press (standing/double leg)	1x10	1-2x8-10	311	2m

Stage 2 : C Day - Exercise Descriptions

Here are descriptions of the exercises involved in C day, Stage 2 of the *Get Buffed!* ™ II (Get More Buffed!) four (4) stage program.

Squat – MS/MB : Now that you are starting to lift more load in this exercise, it is critical you confirm your technique :

- Face the racks, on which the bar is placed.
- Take hand grip just outside shoulder width, elbows down during the movement.
- Step under the bar, bringing your body to the bar, and evenly position the bar on your back. Then extend your legs and take the load on your back.
- Step back but take only minimum steps necessary.
- Head stays in line with spine throughout so at start look straight or slightly down.
- 'Set' the pelvis by performing a small posterior rotation.
- Initiate descent with concurrent hip and knee action.
- Focus on sucking tummy during lowering.
- Only lower as far as you can without exceeding 45 degree trunk flexion.
- Keep the spine in line with the hips.
- Keep knees even distance apart throughout descent and ascent.
- As you reverse the eccentric phase in a concentric phase focus on driving with gluts.
- Ensure that you 'come up the same way you came down'.
- Avoid hips rising faster than shoulders.
- Upon completion of the set walk forward and rack bar.

When you step backwards out of the racks assume a medium stance (shoulder width or just outside).

As the load comes up, the issues of wearing a belt and or knee wraps will no doubt arise. Unless you have no background experience squatting without a belt, I would not see a need for a belt in this phase. But if you have been belt reliant, closely review your decision to 'burn your belt'! If you do go belt-free and are used to wearing a belt, I strongly recommend you be extremely conservative in your load selection! Now for knee wraps – again I don't see the need for them in this phase, and unlike the belt, there is less risks in going 'cold turkey' i.e. if you have a long history of wearing knee wraps, it will be okay to ditch them now.

But one constant for the knees – I strongly recommend wearing knees sleeves – neoprene-like knee slips that provide no support or stability, but serve to maintain a higher knee joint temperature/maintain knee joint temperature during rest periods.

Squat – NS/HB : As per the above technique, but place the bar higher on the upper back, and assume a slightly narrower than shoulder width stance. The more you want to isolate the quads, the narrower you should go in the stance. Feet together is an option albeit an extreme one, and be prepared to lower the loading the closer together your feet are.

Now the 1.5's technique is used here and I will go over that again. Lower down to the bottom of your range (ideally thigh below parallel to the ground!), pause, then come up 1/3 of the way, pause, then go back down to the bottom, pause, then stand up all the way, but don't fully lock out the knees. This is one rep. Pause in this slightly knee bent position before going again.

Dynamic Lunge : Place the bar on the upper back behind the head ala the squat. Step out with your weakest side leg in front of you, bending both knees in one continual fast movement until the knee of the back leg is almost on the ground. Then without pausing drive back up with the front leg and return to the start position, i.e. with feet side by side. Then go on the other side etc.

Now if you have a significant strength imbalance right to left in this movement, try this unique technique that I have developed. Do two reps on the weak side consecutively, then one on the strong side. Then continue in this pattern. 10 reps a side in a conventional approach becomes a total of 21 reps – 14 on the weak side, 7 on the strong side.

Single Leg Squat : I want you all to do this one single leg, irrespective of your bilateral leg strength balance. Very simple concept – stand on one leg and squat as far down as your strength or flexibility (or both!) will tolerate. I am going to throw in three options – from the easiest to the most challenging.

    a. On a very reclined hack squat.
    b. Leaning back on to a Swiss ball with the ball up against a wall (just need to position the ball appropriately).
    c. Free standing, maybe with a vertical frame nearby to hold for balance.

Generally speaking, I encourage you to pursue range over reps, but initially use a range that allows you to get at least 8 - 10 reps.

Calf Press – standing, double : Using both feet in a standing calf press machine (pads on shoulders), make sure you work through full range – full stretch, full height. If your right to left imbalance in the calf's is significant, consider doing this unilaterally, and perhaps you will need to go back to bodyweight or bodyweight plus a little external loading – sometimes the weight of the calf press (depending upon the design of the one you are using) can be too much for single leg work.

Stage 2, Option 1 – Hypertrophy / Lower Training Age

D Day

Exercise	Warm up	Work	Speed	Rest
Bent over Row (MG/prone)	10/8	6/1/6/1	311	alternate with incline bench
Incline Bench Press (MG)	10/8	6/1/6/1	311	alternate with b/over row
Prone DB Fly	opt 1x10	1x6-8+ 1x6-8+ 1x6-8	311	strip set alternate with dips
Dips	1x10 x b/dips	1-2x8-10	311	alternate with prone fly

Stage 2, Option 2 - Hypertrophy-neural / Intermediate Training Age

D Day

Exercise	Warm up	Work	Speed	Rest
Bent over Row (MG/prone)	10/8	5/1/5/1	311	alternate with incline bench
Incline Bench Press (MG)	10/8	5/1/5/1	311	alternate with b/over row
Prone DB Fly	opt 1x8	1x12-15	311	alternate with dips
Dips	1x8 x b/dips	1-2x6-8	311	alternate with prone fly

Stage 2, Option 3 - Neural/Advanced Training Age

D Day

Exercise	Warm up	Work	Speed	Rest
Bent over Row (MG/prone)	10/8	4/1/4/1 1x10-15	311	alternate with incline bench
Incline Bench Press (MG)	10/8/6	4/1/4/1 1x10-15	311	alternate with b/over row
Standing EZ bar Reverse Bi Curl	1x10	1-2x5-6 Opt 1x10	311	2-3min

Stage 2 : D Day - Exercise Descriptions

Here are descriptions of the exercises involved in D day, Stage 2 of the *Get Buffed!* ™ II (Get More Buffed!) four (4) stage program.

Bent Over Row - MG/L-MB : Stand with your feet shoulder width or slightly wider apart. Bend forward at the waist and push you hips back a bit, so that the center of gravity of your body is as close to directly over the legs as possible. Have the legs slightly bent. Keep the trunk flat in a line or angle slightly above horizontal to the ground, and do not allow this angle to change whatsoever during the lift. Take a medium grip on a barbell and raise it to a low point on your chest. Use a full stretch, and ensure you make it to the trunk. Focus on pulling with the shoulder blades, and squeezing them together at the top.

Now as per some of the other exercises (more so the 'pulling' or flexion movements) there is the temptation to cheat. Aim to resist this but don't be too concerned if it happens slightly in the last few reps, more so in the last week of this stage. However don't risk any back injuries by excessive and or sudden trunk extension.

As the loads increase in this lift, there is a specific way I like to get into position, to reduce the risk of injury and strain on the lower back. I recommend you deadlift the bar off the ground into a standing position, and then lower the bar down, keeping it close to the body as you simultaneously bend the hips and knees towards the final position. If for whatever reason you don't want the work of getting it off the ground to start, you can set the bar up on low blocks or even a prone bench, and step back with the bar, using the same set up after that.

Incline Bench Press – MG/MB : Using an incline bench angle of about 30 degrees, take a medium grip on the bar (medium is with the hands just inside the lines on a standard Olympic type bar), and lower the bar to a medium position on the chest (i.e. roughly in line with the nipples). When you press back up, avoid full lockout. Now a spotter shouldn't be optional here – make it a must do! Remember when fatigue sets in (particularly in the triceps) in this lift, failure can come swiftly and with dire consequences! If you are training with no hope of getting a spotter (e.g. solo) do yourself a favor and use a power rack with the safety racks set just out of range reach, but high enough to prevent you crushing your sternum!

Another need for the spotter is the concern of taking load in the above forehead position, when taking the bar out of or returning it to the racks. This is a position of higher stress on the shoulder and neck joints.

Also, because of the relatively weak position when un-racking/re-racking the bar, you can lose a lot of energy in doing so. So when getting closer to your maximum this alone is a reason to use a spotter that knows also how to 'lift out' – a skill in itself. You need to teach them to lift at your signal, stay with the bar as you move it horizontally towards the starting position, and then release it slowly and evenly back into your control. You don't want them dumping the weight onto you!

How many spotters should you use? Your choices are basically 1, 2 or 3. I would go 1 or 3 only – I don't like having 2. There is too big a risk with 2 - that one will lift earlier or more than the other side lifter – and you can cop a serious injury (e.g. pec tear) from this error. Having a center spotter over your head, which you have in a 1 or 3 spotter situation, negates this to a large extent.

Prone DB Fly : Lie face down on a bench. Keep the elbows only slightly bent and at a constant angle throughout. Raise the arms up to the side, keeping them approx. 90 degrees to the long axis of the body. Pause at top. Do not rest the hands on the floor between reps, and minimize the upper trap involvement.

Cheating is not much of a concern here because it is nearly impossible, but be conscious NOT to arch your upper back or elevate (raise) your upper traps. I want a posturally flat (so called correct) position in which to retract (pull in) the shoulder blades. You may experience some loss in range however, which I would only tolerate in latter reps and weeks within this 3 week cycle.

Dips or Bench Dip : If your triceps are not up to it, do bench dips (between 2 benches). Otherwise, use a medium width (just outside shoulders) parallel bar. Cross the feet at the ankles, bend the knees so the ankles are at or near knee height. Lower down until the shoulders are lower the elbow joint (providing you have no joint or injuries conditions that contraindicate this). Keep the body still during the lift and lower, so the movement is not affected by momentum. Do not lock out fully at the top.

Either way, warm up using bench dips. If you are going to use significant external loading in the work sets, I would also recommend a second warm up set of at least a few reps with body weight.

Now you are hopefully going to use external loading in this exercise in at least one of the work-sets! You can use my method of applying external loading as per outlined for the chin ups if you like.

Note in the Neural/Advanced Training Age Option for the first upper body program in the week, this exercise is performed at the end of B day.

Stage 2 – Concluding Comments

After a fairly light yet painful Stage 1, you will by now realize that Stage 2 of this second generation *Get Buffed!*™ program is not messing around – straight into significantly more loading. Which is why it is a more advanced program than the first generation *Get Buffed!*™ programs. So I say again – if you have not done the original *Get Buffed!*™ program, this second generation program may be too advanced for you. And if you are going to go back and do the original *Get Buffed!*™ program, you may be interested in knowing that you can get the whole program on video – all 16 different workouts (four stages, four different workouts per stage) – with myself demonstrating. You can find out more about these videos by at <u>www.getbuffed.net</u>.

What appeared complex in Stage 1 of this program by virtue of the exercises and loading parameter may now seem simplistic – few exercises, few sets, less variety in loading protocols. However don't mistake simple for being ineffective – just get it done and let the results tell you the answers. A final suggestion – don't look to get strong today. Do in today's workout what is going to make you stronger in the next workout of the same kind!

Stage 3

Stage 3 – Overview

You are halfway through the program – by now you should be noticing some changes. But the best is yet to come! Provided you haven't over-trained, you can expect to see even greater results in size and strength in the second half of this 4-stage program. I have raised two issues in this first paragraph that I want to go back and give further details on.

Firstly my proviso – if you haven't over-trained. Let's qualify this – if you have placed your fatigue in a position on the fatigue/recovery curve where you are below homeostasis (the base line) and have been for some time (and chances are still going south!), then you are less likely to experience the increased adaptations available in this second half of this 4 stage program. At best, you will miss only a small percentage of the potential adaptations. At worst, you will get ill, injured, or just get frustrated and drop out. This is not good!

Whilst ideally I want you making recovery decisions on a daily basis, this halfway mark is one of the more critical moments of recovery decision-making in any 12-week program. An error in this decision can diminish or totally negate the potential gains that should be received in the second half of the program.

So at this half way point let's iron this out. Not only retrospectively, but looking forward. Let's make the decisions now that will ensure you stay in the program and get the maximum out of it! Here we go – should you be taking a rest week now before you get into Stage 3? I hope you have selected a recovery model as outlined earlier in the book – but now I am going to ask you to forget that. Yes, forget your earlier decision. Training is a process, not a prescription. The best approach is to make a plan and modify it daily. So irrespective of what recovery model you initially selected – should you now be modifying it?

How do you know the answer to this question? Here are some helpful questions:

1. Did you feel stronger in every week?
2. Did you remain keen to train in every week?
3. If your goal was to put on weight did it happen?
4. Are you sleeping well?
5. Do you wake up feeling refreshed each morning?

If you answered yes to these five simple questions, I assume your recovery is on track. If you even got so much as one no or a maybe to any of the above, review your recovery model and ask the question 'should I take a recovery week now?' If you answered no to four or more of the above questions, don't even consider training this week!!!

Typically when making this decision as to whether a recovery week is required here, one often makes it based on how you feel now. That is not enough. I want you to make this decision based on a projection into the future, by asking yourself this question *"Based on how I am feeling now, how will I feel in 2-4 wks time if I don't take a recovery week now?"* That is an example of how to project into the future to make decisions for now.

Now asking the question is often only half the equation! It is so tempting for an individual who is answering their own question to over-ride rationale with emotion, ignoring obvious signs of fatigue and pushing on because of fear (of losing shape) and / or greed (want it now!). So bouncing your response off a significant other has merit. For high-level athletes who I work with, I tend to ensure they respect their intuition and rationale, not their emotion! But if you don't have a coach, and if you suspect you have historically over-ruled logic with emotion, bounce your response off a levelheaded person you respect. Let them keep you honest to yourself!

The second point I wanted to address was my earlier comment and your possible confusion: More size? I know what you are thinking – the reps are coming down lower, and the textbook says that you will only put on size in the 6-8 and above bracket. Forget the textbook – listen to your body! I cannot tell you precisely why this increase in size is likely to happen in the second Stage of the program, but I can hypothesize. With my unique approach to program design, you have learnt to recruit more of muscle fiber in the early stages of these programs. Remember – that phase where I told you to learn how to make a light weight create high level fatigue and feel heavy?! That is forcing you to increase your recruitment pattern from one perspective. Then we exploit this enhanced recruitment and add to it by forcing increased recruitment from a loading perspective. Not an exact answer, but a big possibility. In a nutshell, through increased ability to activate all available muscle through retraining in the early stages, we have an increased strength potential and greater size results in the latter stages.

Now what's in store in Stage 3?

The **abdominal program** in this stage continues to progress in level of difficulty. Remember that the rate of change or improvement for any given exercise/action/muscle group may not be the same as another. So treat each abdominal sub-group individually, recognizing that they will not necessarily all move forward at the same rate.

I again encourage you to review the placement of the abdominal exercises in this phase. That is, to ask – should I be doing them at the start or the end of the workout? What I said earlier in the book was that the traditional approach has been to do the abdominal training at the end of the workout. That somewhere along the way someone came up with a paradigm that executing abdominal training early in the workout would cause increased injury potential due to weakened stabilizers. As you would know from reading that discussion, I don't buy into that paradigm. I went on to say that in Stages 1 and 2, if you were lacking in the abdominal strength and control, I would expect the abs to appear first in the workout. However, in Stages 3 and 4, <u>provided</u> you have achieved your minimal abdominal standards, you could move them to the back of the workout.

We are now at a point where I raise that question for you to answer – should you, in Stage 3, be performing the abdominal exercises at the start or end of the workout? To help you answer this, simply compare your current position or ability in the abdominals relative to your current position/ability in the exercises that make up the balance of your workout. Whatever is lagging should be done first!

The **upper body program** dominates over the lower body in Stages 3 and 4 if you use a linear periodization, and in Stages 2 and 4 if you use an alternating approach. In Stage 3 pushing dominates over pulling. This is so because the first exercise on the first workout of the week is bench press.

Note this is the first time that bench press has appeared as high as this in the week's sequence of exercise in all the stages so far. I de-emphasize bench for a while in an attempt to return some balance to the average weight trainers bodies, after training career habits of doing bench first in the workout, in the first upper body workout of the week, ALL THE TIME! Hopefully by now the upper back is stronger and the anterior muscles of the upper torso are longer, more able to contract! And will make a massive contribution to a bigger bench press! Something that you may have doubted would result when you did the first Stage and noted the bench was virtually done last in the workout on the last day upper body day of the week! If you had the faith to stick to my plan (as crazy as it may have seemed to you at the time) you will be rewarded!

If you are following the linear periodization plan you will be going lower in reps and doing less exercises in this stage compared to Stage 2. If you are going to work the alternating plan, you will be using this program after Stage 1 and then doing Stage 2 after this stage (which means you may not have been able to advance too much in the program till getting this stage!). There is an eccentric set in all versions (hypertrophy, mixed, and neural), and pushing and pulling are mixed on both workout days.

As noted above, this program is based on alternate setting. This method has been fully explained earlier in the book. If your gym is busy and it is difficult to alternate between two work stations without needing your own guards to retain the equipment, just take a normal standard set rest approach e.g. set, rest, repeat set of same exercise, rest, repeat set of same exercise etc. until all sets for that exercise are complete.

And make sure you use spotters whenever the load is above the body, and especially good ones for the eccentric sets! I want you to refer to the section just below in this section, where I give further information on eccentric training, to ensure you perform these movements safely and effectively.

In the **lower body** training, we are going to return to quad dominant i.e. quad dominant exercises will occur first in the training week. If you are following the linear periodization plan you will be going lower in reps. If you are going to work the alternating plan, you will be using this program after Stage 1 and then doing Stage 2 after this stage (Stage 3). The number of exercises per workout is less in this stage than in Stage 2, and the sequence of exercise in each workout is big muscle group exercise to small. And there is an eccentric set in all versions (hypertrophy, mixed, and neural).

Finally, you will see that the leg workouts have been changed from the first and third workout of the week in Stages 1 and 2, to being the second and fourth workouts of the week in Stage 4.

The following provides **general information about this stage of the program**:

Note that the 6/5/4 or 5/4/3 or 4/3/2 loading model is used in this phase. These are called waves (some call them pyramids) are based on the following concept – as you lower the rep into the next set, you raise the weight. The key is in selecting the correct weight, and I strongly discourage going too close to your maximum early, or you may find in the subsequent set you are not able to achieve the target reps with a slightly heavier load.

The critical key to load selection in wave loading is to avoid total fatigue off any of the early sets. For example, if the first work set in a wave was 5 reps, I don't recommend doing a 100% or your 5RM (repetition maximum). Rather, about 90%. So in lay terms, at the 5th rep you might still have another rep in you, but of course you don't do it! If you don't respect this you may negate the potential neural 'dis-inhibition' that wave loading offers!

The increments from set to set can be considered as percentages rather than a raw score. For example, 1.25 kg increment in a bicep curl may seem small, but it may be the same as a 10 kg increment in a squat. Both would be 5% jumps if the prior work sets were 25 kgs in the bicep curl and 200 kgs in the squat.

Sample loading pattern in week 1 for the 6/5/4 + 1x 4 eccentric method:

1 x 6 @ 100 kg

1 x 5 @ 110 kg

1 x 4 @ 120 kg

1 x 4 @ 140 kg

Then in the next week, see below:

Sample loading pattern in week 2 for the 6/5/4 + 1x4 eccentric method:

1 x 6 @ 105 or 110 kg

1 x 5 @ 115 or 120 kg

1 x 4 @ 125 or 130 kg

1 x 4 @ 145 or 150 kg

Of course, if there is a third week, the same technique applies but the increments don't need to be as high.

Eccentric Set Guidelines

I have also added an eccentric set to the entire upper body program at the end of these single waves (they are called single waves because they are not repeated again in that workout in the same exercise). I want to take time here to ensure you know how to perform eccentric sets <u>safely</u> and <u>effectively.</u>

The eccentric set requires you to lower under control a load you could not lift – possibly somewhere between 10-25% more than your RM for that number of reps. RM is the maximum load you can lift for the number of reps required. You will also need to have an appropriately trained partner/s doing the work in the lifting phase of the eccentric set. The critical key in load selection for the eccentric set is to select a load that you can control at the desired speed (in this program, this ranges from a 5 to 3 second eccentric time frame, and that does not overload any injury potential you may have. Eccentric training, by virtue of going closer to your limit, has inherent higher risk. I recommend you do NOT do this set if you have any potential for injury, or if you don't have adequately trained spotters!

For example, if you feel you are up to doing eccentric squats, you could do them instead of the ¼ or bench squats that shown in this program. However I believe the number of people that can safely eccentric squat are lower than the number who can say safely eccentric bench, so in the program I have placed an overload movement (1/4 squat, deadlift off blocks) to replace the eccentric lifts in the lower body.

Safety is my main concern. I have included overload (supra-maximal load options) because as one becomes more advanced they are a necessary part of training to exploit your potential. If you do decide to do eccentric squats, I strongly advice they be performed only by :

- Intermediate and advanced lifters.

- And only when there are experienced competent, focused, spotters on hand who are physically capable of managing the load.

- And you are not injured or feeling any slight niggles in the joints or muscles directly or indirectly involved.

Bottom line – eccentric overload presents higher injury risk – <u>if in doubt don't do eccentric sets!</u>

Back-off Set Guidelines

The key in the back-off set is to select a load that allows you not only to do the reps required, but allows you to rehearse and experience 'speed' in the concentric phase. By this I mean I want you to aim to lift as fast as you can, and to 'feel' the higher speed of movement.

Sample loading pattern in week 1 for the 5/4/3/3ECC/12-15 method:

1 x 5 @ 100 kg

1 x 4 @ 105 kg

1 x 3 @ 110 kg

1 x 3 @ 130 kg ECC

1x 12 @ 80 kgs

Sample loading pattern in week 2 for the 5/4/3/3ECC/12-15 method:

1 x 5 @ 102.5 kg

1 x 4 @ 107.5 kg

1 x 3 @ 112.5 kg

1 x 3 @ 132.5 kg ECC

1x 13 @ 80 kgs

Sample loading pattern in week 3 for the 5/4/3/3ECC/12-15 method:

1 x 5 @ 105 kg

1 x 4 @ 110 kg

1 x 3 @ 115 kg

1 x 3 @ 135 kg ECC

1x 14 @ 80 kgs

Now go and *Get Buffed!*™

Stage 3 – Warm Up / Stretching / Abdominal / Control Drills

A & C Day

Exercise	Warm up	Work	Speed	Rest
Warm Up	optional 5-15 minutes of light aerobic type activity e.g. stationary bike			
Stretch	10-20 minutes of upper body stretching			
Abdominals				
Knee up vertical	15 on incline*	1-2x5-15	311	1-2m
Modified V-sits	15 at b/wgt*	1-2x5-15 With ext load	311	1-2m
Side raises + twist on Roman Chair	10/side at b/wgt*	1-2x5-15 per side	311	1-2m
Control Drills				
Flutters	nil	1x10-15	202	0-30s
Scarecrow	nil	1x 10	202	0-30s
Side Lying Ext DB Rotation	nil	1x10-15	202	0-30s
Prone Limited Range DB Row	nil	1x10-15	202	0-30s

Workout

---

* only need to do a warm up set if you plan to use external resistance in the work sets. If you don't plan to use external resistance in the work sets, ignore warm up set.

Stage 3 : A & C Day – Abdominal Exercise Descriptions

Here are descriptions of the abdominal exercises involved in A and C day, Stage 3 of the *Get Buffed!* ™ II (Get More Buffed!) four (4) stage program.

Knee Up on vertical : If in the prior stage you chose to perform this exercise on the flat (lying back on ground) then you should progress to the incline version (as described in the prior stage). If you were doing the incline version of this exercise last time, you should look to do the vertical version in this stage.

There are a number of options you can chose from to perform the vertical knee up variation. These include :

i.   Hanging from a chin bar, gripping shoulder width with palms facing in the direction you are facing; or

ii.   Supporting your body on your lower arms on a frame designed specifically for this exercise (lower arms are parallel to the ground); or

iii.   Hands through straps that hang down from supports above.

No matter which device you choose, the guidelines remain constant. In the first instance start the movement with the knees and hips at ninety degrees. Keep them at these joint angles throughout the movement. Then lift the knees to the chest, bringing them as close to the chest as you can. This will involve the lower back rounding.

The greatest challenge you face in this movement (apart from the obvious of lifting the knees to the chest) is to lift and lower the legs within minimal or no body sway. The technique I recommend is to lift your legs in a smooth, controlled, non-accelerated method. Then pause them at the top. And then lower them taking three seconds. Using this controlled method will minimize the body sway. It will also reduce the number of reps you can do!

Now for whatever reason you need more resistance (I don't think this will apply to too many people!) here are two progressively harder options :

a. Start with your legs full extended, and as you lift (flex your hip) bring you knees up to your chest by bending also at the knees; lower back in reverse i.e. extending your legs out as you lower down.

b. For an even higher level of difficulty, start with your legs straight and lift them up keeping the straight at all times. Lower them down in a mirror image of this i.e. keeping them straight at all times.

This is one lift I strongly suggest you be smart about. It is possibly the abdominal exercise that places the most strength on the lower back, through the pull of the hip flexors. So this is no time to aim to impress the audience. Just stick with what you can do well.   And if you experience lower back discomfort, look for a lower level of difficulty option!

From a purists point of view your pelvis should remain at a constant angle throughout, rather than rolling forward from the top (anterior rotation) during the most difficult ranges. However my coaching philosophy is to drill you in lead up movements such that this control happens automatically, rather than attempt to coach or have you cue yourself during more complex movements.   I see so many times coaches/trainers cueing finer points during a complex lift and for the most part they are wasting their time. If it isn't happening by itself, I usually go back to a lower level of difficulty and progress back up.

I also want to share another teaching philosophy I use – that as the level of difficulty rises, I don't demand the same level of 'perfection' technically. Rather, I allow some drop off. Not to the extent that the person's health is at risk or where we are departing so much from our initial position it would raise the question *'why did we have that initial technical focus?'* Not that far. But a more relaxed view on technique. And then whatever less than perfect occurred, we aim to perform at a higher level technically the next time we progress up through the technical focus to this more loaded phase.

Notes :

Speed of movement – Controlled dynamic movement at 313.

Selecting appropriate level - Start conservatively in your load selection, and progress over the subsequent workouts and weeks; ensure that no inappropriate loading is being experienced in the lower back (lumbar).

Modified V-sits : Lie on your back on the ground. You are going to flex (lift) the hips/legs and trunk at the same time. The end goal is to be in the nearly full seated position with the thighs close to the chest. Your body will create a V shape at the top, with the trunk leaning back about 45-60 degrees and your upper legs forming this angle also. Just imagine your trunk and thighs creating a V-shape.

As your legs lift, bend your knees and aim the knees towards the chest. Lift the legs at the same rate as the trunk i.e. don't get one ahead of the other! This lift can be a challenge from a co-ordination perspective, but mastery of this is rewarding!

As you flex the hip/legs and trunk simultaneously, your arms will raise but keep them parallel to the ground at all times. If you want to make it even harder, when you lower down to the bottom position, do not allow your heels or upper back or arms to rest on the ground!

As with the knee ups, this exercise can place considerable strain through the hip flexors, so ensure that you are not aggravating the lower back in any way by performing this movement.

The pull of the hip flexors should be countered to some extent by the pelvis rolling backwards (posterior rotation) as your trunk flexes up.

Now should you require an increased resistance (which I don't believe will apply to many of you) you can place a weight plate on your chest, holding it with your arms crossed over your chest like an 'X'.

Notes :

Speed of movement – Controlled dynamic movement at 313.

Selecting appropriate level - start conservatively in your load selection, and progress over the subsequent workouts and weeks; ensure that no inappropriate loading is being experienced in the lower back (lumbar); your choose in load selection is to place weight plates on your chest.

Side Raises plus Twist on Roman Chair : You will have been performing the basis of this variation in the previous stage. To refresh your memory, I will describe it again.

Lie on your side on a bench or a device known as the Roman Chair. The bench or Roman Chair supports your hips and legs, and your trunk is off the bench. In the case of a normal bench, you will need someone to hold your feet. In the case of the Roman Chair, hook your feet under the heel pad. Lower the body down, maintaining this sideways position. Go as far down as is safe and comfortable, and return to the starting position.

The variation I am applying for this stage is that as you flex upwards, begin progressively rotating your trunk until you are as faced upwards to the roof as much as you can at the top position. As you lower the trunk down, you simply reverse this rotation till you get back sideways towards the bottom half of the lowering.

As I explained in the prior stage, the placement of the hands will alter the level of difficulty. The further the hands are above the head, the harder the movement. In the initial position, I suggest you cross the arms on the chest. Options for increased resistance include :

a. Placing the arms on the head, touching the front of the forehead, elbows angled in at 45 degrees.
b. Placing the arms on the head, touching the back of the forehead, elbows angled out at 90 degrees from the head (so the arms form a straight line from one arm to the next.
c. Extending the arms over the head.
d. Placement of external resistance (e.g. weight plate, med ball etc) on the chest.

Notes :

Speed of movement – A controlled lift, say a speed of 311 or 211.

Arm positions - Start with arms crossed on chest but take out further above the head or hold a weight plate on the chest as is needed to provide appropriate loading.

Selecting appropriate level – Trial and error.

Stage 3 – Warm Up / Stretching / Abdominal / Control Drills

B & D Day

Exercise	Warm up	Work	Speed	Rest
Warm Up	10-20 minutes of light aerobic type activity e.g. stationary bike			
Stretch	20-40 minutes of lower body stretching			
Abdominals				
Curl up with load	15 at b/wgt*	1-2x10-20	201	1-2m
Wrist to Knee Curl Up	15 at b/wgt*	1-2x10-20	201	1-2m
Extended body holds	nil	1-2x30-120s	30-120s holds	1-2m
Control Drills				
Light leg extensions	nil	1x10-15	202	0-30s
Prone lying single leg hip / thigh extensions	nil	1x10-15	202	0-30s
Side Lying Lateral Leg Raise	nil	1x10-15	202	0-30s
Co-Contraction Lunge	nil	1x10-20	202	0-30s
Lying Supine Single Leg Hip/Thigh Extension	nil	1x5-10	202	0-30s
Assisted Squat	nil	1x10	202	0-30s
Workout				

* only need to do a warm up set if you plan to use external resistance in the work sets. If you don't plan to use external resistance in the work sets, ignore warm up set.

Stage 3 : B & D Day – Abdominal Exercise Descriptions

Here are descriptions of the abdominal exercises involved in B and D day, Stage 3 of the *Get Buffed!* ™ II (Get More Buffed!) four (4) stage program.

Curl Up with load : This is the same body position that I have had you use throughout in the curl up - lying on your back on the ground, knees bent to about 90 degrees, and feet flat on the floor. Your feet are not to be anchored under anything. Then you sit up or curl up the trunk, ideally to a full sitting position.

In this stage however I want you to hold a weight plate on your chest. Start out with a very light one!!!

If you plan on using external load (weight on the chest) in the work sets, do a bodyweight set to warm up first.

Like any loaded strength training exercise, if you lose the ability to complete the range you used on the first rep, terminate the set.

Notes :

Speed of movement – Attempt to explode up, realizing that the load may have it not looking as fast as your attempt, and then control down. No pause needed.

Arm positions – Assuming you are up to it, the arms will be across the chest holding on to the external loading.

Selecting appropriate level – Trial and error.

Wrist to Knee Curl Ups : Lie on your back on the ground, each hand touching it's own side of the forehead with the fingers, elbows out at 45 degrees. The elbow angle is not to change during the exercise. Starting with legs out straight, raise (flex) the trunk and one leg simultaneously. As you continue into the flexion, rotate the trunk so that the elbow (or preferably the wrist) on the opposite side to the knee that has been lifted touches the opposite knee. Then return to fully straight body position, repeating next rep on other side.

If you did need to add resistance, you can hold weight on your chest (or add light angle weights, or both). This would mean you would not be touching wrist to opposite knee, rather looking to bring the knee as close as you can to the opposite side of the chest/shoulder.

Notes :

Speed of movement – Perform this movement explosively during the lift, and then control down. No pause needed.

Arm positions - Have the fingers lightly touching the front of the head, elbow out at 45 degrees from the body, and arm/elbow angle not changing during the lift. The placement of the hands will alter the level of difficulty. The further the hands are above the head, the harder the movement.

Extended Body Holds : Place your feet on a bench and your elbows on a Swiss ball or another bench out in front of you. Rest your elbows on the ball or bench, so that you are extended out as far as you can hold. What I mean by this is, with your elbows on the ball or bench, if you slid that out further (so that your elbows are further out in front of you as opposed to being under your chest), what would be the most extreme point you could hold? Once in that position, hold it for as long as you can. If you do exceed 2 minutes (and I don't expect you will), and you are not able to safely extend your arms out further, have someone place a medicine ball or weight plate on your hips or lower back.

Notes :

Speed of movement – Hold each extended position for somewhere between 30 and 120 seconds. If you cannot hold the position for at least 30 seconds, look to make the position easier by bringing your elbows under your body – not during the movement ideally, but prior to starting the hold. How to make it harder, should you reach the 2 minute mark, is described above.

Arm positions - Start with the elbows under the shoulders, shoulder width or inside shoulder width. Extend the elbows forward to make it harder.

Stage 3, Option 1 - Hypertrophy / Lower Training Age

A Day

Exercise	Warm up	Work	Speed	Rest
Bench Press	10/8/6	6/5/4	211	alternate
(MG/LB/FD/Med arch)		1x4	500	with
		1x15-20	211	bicep curl
Bicep Curl	10/8/6	6/5/4	211	alternate
(EZ/PB/supine grip)		1x4	500	with
		1x15-20	211	bench press

Stage 3, Option 2 - Hypertrophy-neural / Intermediate Training Age

A Day

Exercise	Warm up	Work	Speed	Rest
Bench Press	10/8/5	5/4/3	211	alternate
(MG/LB/FD/Med arch)		1x3	500	with
		1x12-15	211	bicep curl
Bicep Curl	10/8/5	5/4/3	211	alternate
(EZ/PB/supine grip)		1x3	500	with
		1x12-15	211	bench press

Stage 3, Option 3 - Neural/Advanced Training Age

A Day

Exercise	Warm up	Work	Speed	Rest
Bench Press (MG/LB/FD/ Med arch)	10/8/5 with opt 1x3	4/3/2 1x2 1x10-12	211 400 211	alternate with bicep curl
Bicep Curl (EZ/PB/supine grip)	10/8/5 opt 1x3	4/3/2 1x2 1x10-12	211 400 211	alternate with bench press

Stage 3 : A Day - Exercise Descriptions

Here are descriptions of the exercises involved in A day, Stage 3 of the *Get Buffed!* ™ II (Get More Buffed!) four (4) stage program.

Bench Press : (medium grip, low bar, feet down, medium arch) Take a medium grip on the bench press. For most this will be with the little fingers inside the lines on the Olympic bar. You will lower the bar down to the lower portion of the chest - this is a strong position, allowing a greater arc in the bar movement and greater lat involvement. Your feet are to be on the ground.

I want you to use what I call a medium arch. The simple concept of an arch is to bring the hips and shoulders closer together, creating a bow like effect in the trunk. This reduces the distance of travel for the bar, and again increases the contribution of the lats. There are a number of ways to get into this position, and here is one. Once you have established your grip and your upper back position on the bench, move you legs up a bit further, to an acute knee angle. This will allow you to lift or slide your hips closer to your head, resulting in a arch of the spine. In the final position, your feet should be flat and pointed slightly outward, knee angle acute (less then 90 degrees), bum, upper back and head in constant contact with the bench, legs tight and butt cheeks squeezed (resulting in increased force into ground through the feet).

Note the greater the arch, potentially the heavier the loads you can lift, but I don't want the maximum arch you can attain in this program – save this for Stage 4.

If you want a visual display/discussion of arching in the bench, you can find it in my *Ian King's Guide to the Bench Press* video or find an experienced powerlifter to give you some tips.

A few tips regarding benching as the load is increased :

- Use chalk on the hands to prevent outward slipping.
- Use wrist wraps to reduce strain on the wrist joint.
- If the bench is high for you (short legs or unusually high bench) place a plate on the ground under each foot (45 cm off the ground is standard bench press bench height).
- Check the bar is not bent before starting. Even a slight bend can reduce ability to lift high loads and increase injury potential.
- Use spotters for all work sets.
- Consider a lift off and rack for the heaviest sets, and have the spotter and you rehearse this in a prior set.
- Do not allow the feet to slip or move from their starting position, and keep the bum down!

I stress again only do the eccentric bench set if you are experienced, injury free and have experienced spotters. If there is any risk of injury, pass up this option. Just delete the set.

Remember - the bench is to be alternated with the bicep curl using a full recovery alternated set method.

Bicep Curl : (medium grip, EZ curl bar, standing) Take a medium grip on the EZ bar, so that your hands are slightly internally rotated. If you want to save lifting the bar off the ground each time, sit it on a bench or similar. The starting position is with the arms by the side. As you lift, aim to slide the elbows back a bit, and leave them there for the duration of the lift. Bend the elbows to the point where to take the bar any higher, the elbows would have to come forward, then lower from there. Make sure you do go to full extension at the end of the eccentric phase. Whilst I am sure there are specific hypertrophy benefits from not fully extending, I don't like the thought of altering (shortening) the length of the biceps too much, which I believe may occur from chronic use of non-full extension in bicep curling.

You may also want to stand with you feet shoulder width apart, knees slightly bent. Maintaining this knee position can help minimize or prevent extension through the spine. I am not as concerned about injury from this (which I believe has been blown out of proportion) but rather I want to isolate the action to elbow flexion, not elbow flexion plus shoulder flexion plus trunk extension etc – with the intent of isolating the work to the forearm flexors.

I do believe that the tendency to and the benefits from using cheat movements is greater in flexion (pulling) movements than extension movements (pushing), or at least these benefits apply earlier in the strength capacity of these lifts. This is a discussion in itself but I suspect it may be tied to the weaker force curves typically evident in many joint flexions. What I am saying is I allow cheating earlier in flexion movements (e.g. biceps) than extension movements (e.g. bench press)!

Stage 3, Option 1 - Hypertrophy / Lower Training Age

B Day

Exercise	Warm up	Work	Speed	Rest
Squat (LB/MS)	1x10/1x8/	1x6 1x6 1x5 1x4	301	3-4m
¼ Squat (or box squat) LB/MS	nil	1-2x4	201	3-4m
Squat (MB/MS)	nil	1x10	301	2-3m
Squat (HB/NS)	nil	1x15-20	301	2m
Jump Lunge	10/leg	10/leg	10*	1-2m
OR				
Jump Squat	1x10	1x10	10*	1-2m

Stage 3, Option 2 - Hypertrophy-neural / Intermediate Training Age

B Day

Exercise	Warm up	Work	Speed	Rest
Squat (LB/MS)	1x10/1x8/	1x5 1x5 1x4 1x3	301	4-5m
¼ Squat (or box squat) LB/MS	nil	1-2x3	201	4-5m
Squat (MB/MS)	nil	1x8	301	3-4m
Squat (HB/NS)	nil	1x12-15	301	3m
Jump Lunge	8/leg	8/leg	10*	2-3m
OR				
Jump Squat	1x8	1x8	10*	2-3m

Stage 3, Option 3 - Neural/Advanced Training Age

B Day

Exercise	Warm up	Work	Speed	Rest
Squat (LB/MS)	1x10/1x8/	1x4 1x5 1x3 1x2	301	5m
¼ Squat (or box squat) LB/MS	nil	1-2x2	201	5m
Squat (MB/MS)	nil	1x5	301	4-5m
Squat (HB/NS)	nil	1x8	301	4m
Jump Lunge	6/leg	6/leg	10*	3m
OR				
Jump Squat	1x6	1x6	10*	3m

Stage 3 : B Day - Exercise Descriptions

Here are descriptions of the exercises involved in B day, Stage 3 of the *Get Buffed!* ™ II (Get More Buffed!) four (4) stage program.

Squat – LB/MS : With the bar on a squat rack, approach the bar and place the bar on a low bar height on the shoulders behind the head. What is low bar? Any lower and it would fall off is one way of describing it! Another is to say a bit lower than last stage (e.g. ½ to 1"). Another way is to teach you how to identify 3 different practical and safe heights for the bar on your upper back – I trust you used the highest position in Stage 1, the medium position in Stage 2, and now we are going to use all three in this stage!

When you step backwards out of the racks assume a medium stance (shoulder width or just outside). Confirm your technique as per the description provided earlier.

As the load is being raised even more, the issues of wearing a belt and or knee wraps will no doubt arise. If you plan to use a heavy or thigh powerlifting belt (6") in Stage 4, I would suggest going with a light or thin (4") belt in this phase. I would expect this would apply more so to the neural/advanced lifter than the hypertrophy/beginner program option.

The same applies to knee wraps – if you plan training in Stage 4 with tight knee wraps, use them loose and pulled easy (i.e. not on maximum tightness) in this phase. As with the belt, this should be more of a consideration for the neural/advanced lifter than the hypertrophy/beginner program option.

I want to make it clear that neither belts nor knee wraps are required, but they are options.

¼ **Squat or Bench Squat :** This is here to expose you to supra-maximal loading, a method not only appropriate to the more advanced lifter, but a necessity if you are to exploit your strength potential. This lift is a safer option than a full range eccentric squat, but as discussed above, should you feel that you and your spotters are up to doing a full range eccentric squat, you could do that instead of the ¼ squat.

With the ¼ squat, using a bench to dictate squat depth is an option. Don't use it for safety however if you have a power rack. A power rack would be a better safety option in the absence of spotters, with the pin height adjusted to your desired depth.

Don't feel you need to have power-racks or a bench to give depth feedback. There are many occasions where I prefer you learn the proprioception of what joint angle you are at with the use of external feedback.

But from a safety perspective, you MUST HAVE either great spotters capable of recovering you and the load involved or a safety rack to exit gracefully and safely from any missed reps.

When doing a limited range squat in the absence of safety rack or bench feedback for height, I strongly recommend using a conservative range, to allow you to get a feel for what range you can accommodate with that weight.

You are looking to use a load that you could not at this stage do a full range squat with. But at the risk of repeating myself and in the interests of safety, use a weight you can come up with from the range involved (1/4 – 1/3 the way down) and complete the desired number of reps!

I have allowed up to 2 work sets at this lift but one set will suffice most. If you are going with 2 sets, you have the option of using step loading – going slightly heavier on the second set.

Squat - MB/MS : You are going to go back down in load and do a set with a rep number just above your first work set reps. You are also going to raise the bar back up the upper back/neck to the medium bar position. Now ideally, if your load selection has been smart and you have not induced too much fatigue, you may be able to perform the requested reps at or just below the load you used in the first work set. Now this is despite it being a medium bar position, a potentially weaker squat position.

But don't be discouraged if you cannot maintain the exact load as you did in the first work set. If possible, stay fairly close. But forget ideals – use your technical and strength levels as a guide – you must use a load that allows you to maintain technique within the desired parameters. Now if you haven't had the benefit of me teaching you how to squat personally at a seminar, or seen one of my videos on how to squat (such as Killer Leg Exercises available at www.t-mag.com) then you will need to do your best by reading the link provided above to a description of how I want you to squat.

Squat - HB/NS : Now we are going to go even lighter and place the bar higher, taking a narrower stance. Yes, I have made it hard! And if you were wearing a belt, unless you have some sort of physical dependency, ditch it for this set. Suck the air in deep and just do it! Yes, it is going to hurt doing this high rep set but isn't that self-inflicted pain a beautiful thing!......

Jump Lunge or **Jump Squat :** You have a choice here – one is a bilateral movement, the other is a unilateral movement. There are specific adaptations from either, so just choose one – don't do both!

The jump lunge is like a dynamic lunge (described last stage) but once the back knee is nearly on the ground, you explode up such that you leave the ground and swap the legs – back foot to forward foot and vice versa. When you land on the ground you land in the alternate lunge position and you continue downward until the back knee is almost on the ground etc.

If you are able to use weight, whether you hold DBs in your arms (hanging beside the body) or have a bar on your back is up to you. You will notice you can go heavier but slower or lighter and faster. This is again your decision, influenced mainly by what you want out of it – if you have a speed or power requirement, I would suggest go light and fast. Going light may mean as light as bodyweight only. As this is the last exercise, the outcome is one I could watch all day long!!!

Now for the Jump squat. With a very light load (again either DB in the hands or bar on the back), jump as high as you can and upon landing go immediately down, decelerating only enough to control the end of the lowering phase and where you reverse the movement, and immediately jump for height. With the speed vs. load choice, my suggestion to you is as per the above paragraph. Don't worry too much about loading. The rapid eccentric contraction should be enough to give you that muscle damage you are pursuing!

Stage 3, Option 1 - Hypertrophy / Lower Training Age

C Day

Exercise	Warm up	Work	Speed	Rest
Chin Up (MG/prone)	10/8/6	6/5/4 1x4 1x15-20	211 500 211	alternate with CGBP
Close Grip Bench Press (shoulder width grip)	10/8/6	6/5/4 1x4 1x15-20	211 500 211	alternate with chin up

Stage 3, Option 2 - Hypertrophy-neural / Intermediate Training Age

C Day

Exercise	Warm up	Work	Speed	Rest
Chin Up (MG/prone)	10/8/5	5/4/3 1x3 1x12-15	211 400 211	alternate with CGBP
Close Grip Bench Press (shoulder width grip)	10/8/5	5/4/3 1x3 1x12-15	211 400 211	alternate with chin up

Stage 3, Option 3 - Neural/Advanced Training Age

C Day

Exercise	Warm up	Work	Speed	Rest
Chin Up (MG/prone)	10/8/5	4/3/2	211	alternate
	opt 1x3	1x2	400	with
		1x10-12	211	CGBP
Close Grip Bench Press (shoulder width grip)	10/8/5	4/3/2	211	alternate
	opt 1x3	1x2	400	with
		1x10-12	211	chin up

Stage 3 : C Day - Exercise Descriptions

Here are descriptions of the exercises involved in C day, Stage 3 of the *Get Buffed!* ™ II (Get More Buffed!) four (4) stage program.

Chin Up : (prone/medium grip, i.e. palms facing away grip, shoulder width). Take a shoulder width grip with palms facing away from you. Allow the feet to come off the ground slowly, without inducing any body sway. Cross the feet at the ankle and tuck them up behind you. Pull straight up and finish the pull with the chin over the handgrip level. Don't do another rep if this pulling range is not met.

A key to avoid swaying in the chin up is to control the lowering (eccentric phase) and prevent any body sway during the lowering. Swaying in the chin up is a catch-22 situation. It can help get you a rep or two, but the energy lost in combating the swaying can cost you more, so I recommend using a controlled technique.

As with any exercise I like to isolate the target muscles, and therefore the joint actions. Flexing at the hips and knees and other 'additional' body movements are not uncommon during the concentric phase of the chin, but I discourage them. If you cannot do the rep using the target muscles, don't do the rep. Another concern regarding the use of 'additional' movement of the body to achieve reps is the likelihood of controlling this variable. As the load is increased, if the 'cheating movements' are increased, have you really placed the full additional load through the target muscles? I doubt it.

Here are some more tips for the chin up :

- Use the lat pulldown to warm up on, using the same grip. Your warm up loads are selected as a percentage of your first work set weight.

- If the grip on the chin bar is slippery, use chalk on the hands (only use wrist straps as a last resort).
- I prefer a chin bar that is a continual bar as opposed to 2 ends, as it allows you greater flexibility in choosing your grip position.
- Again I prefer a bar that is straight as opposed to one where the ends dips downwards. If you have to use a bar that dips down at each end, look for one that has the least downward angle. I am not convinced about the mechanics of the bars with excessive downward slope, including the ability to pull the chin over the grip level.
- When using external loading to increase the load, use a method that negates body sway caused by the additional external loading.
- When performing eccentric chins, either have a partner lift you or in the absence of a partner, place a bench under the chin bar and jump up from there, providing it doesn't interfere with your ability to lower.
- Don't start a chin rep unless you know you will finish it.
- In the back off set, really aim for speed in the lift!

The final set of chin is something that I imagine may be concerning you! Relax! If you cannot get at least half the suggested number for the back off set, use the lat pulldown instead. Or use the lat pulldown in a superset to compliment the reps if you don't hit the target on the chin bar. Either way, show speed in the lift!

Close Grip Bench Press : (shoulder width grip, feet down, medium arch). The set up for this is exactly as per the bench press in A day, only on this day take a grip that is above or just outside your shoulders. If you are experiencing wrist discomfort, (in addition to using wrist wraps) you can rotate your hands with the thumbs going outwards, joining your fingers.

All the keys and tips from the bench press above apply here also. You may find you are able to lift within about 5-10% of your conventional bench, usually on the lower side, unless you have above average arm (tricep) strength.

A very important safety comment – if you do fail during a rep on the close grip bench press, it will happen with greater suddenness than the conventional bench press. Don't put yourself through this unpleasant experience! Make sure you use an experienced and trustworthy spotter!

Stage 3, Option 1 - Hypertrophy / Lower Training Age

D Day

Exercise	Warm up	Work	Speed	Rest
Deadlift (MG/O-hand/OG)	1x10 / 1x8 1x6	1x6 1x5 1x4	311	3-4m
	NB can reverse grip if need to			
Deadlift (MG/OB)	nil or 1x4	1-2x4	311	3-4m
	i.e. plates on low blocks, bar starts high shin			
Deadlift (MG/OG)	nil	1x6-8	311	
Deadlift (MG/O-hand/SOB) i.e. stand on 1 2" plate	nil or 1x6	1x10	311	2 m
MG Stiff leg deadlift (round over)	1x6	1x10	311	2m

Stage 3, Option 2 - Hypertrophy-neural / Intermediate Training Age

D Day

Exercise	Warm up	Work	Speed	Rest
Deadlift (MG/O-hand/OG)	1x10 / 1x8 1x5	1x5 1x4 1x3	311	4-5m
Note: can reverse grip if need to				
Deadlift (MG/OB) i.e. plates on low blocks, bar starts high shin	nil or 1x4	1-2x3	311	4-5m
Deadlift (MG/OG)	nil	1x5-8	311	4m
Deadlift (MG/O-hand/SOB) i.e. stand on 1 2" plate	nil or 1x6	1x10	311	3-4 m
MG Stiff legged Deadlift (can round over)	1x4	1x8	3m	

Stage 3, Option 3 - Neural/Advanced Training Age

D Day

Exercise	Warm up	Work	Speed	Rest
Deadlift (MG/O-hand/OG)	1x10 / 1x8 1x6/1x4	1x4 1x3 1x2	311	5m
NB can reverse grip if need to				
Deadlift (MG/OB) i.e. plates on low blocks, bar starts high shin	nil or 1x2	1-2x2	311	5m
Deadlift (MG/O)	nil	1x4-6	311	4m
Deadlift (MG/O-hand/SOB) i.e. stand on 1 2" plate	nil or 1x5	1x5	311	3-4 m
MG S-leg D/lift (can round over)	1x4	1x6	311	3m

Stage 3 : D Day - Exercise Descriptions

Here are descriptions of the exercises involved in D day, Stage 3 of the *Get Buffed!* ™ II (Get More Buffed!) four (4) stage program.

Deadlifts – MG/OG : Using a medium (just outside your legs), palm over grip, and starting from the bottom position, weight rested on the ground. It is critical you confirm your technique as per my recommendations for this lift.

One of the biggest issues to be raised in this exercise at this stage is whether to reverse grip i.e. palms facing opposite direction. If you plan to reverse grip in Stage 4, or are a competitive deadlifter, you should consider reverse gripping in this stage.

Whether you are reverse gripping or not, you will want to use chalk to increase grip retention. I would only recommend wrist straps (that anchor your grip to the bar) as a last option.

The question of whether to use a belt will also come up in relation to this lift. I answer it in the same way I did for the squat in Stage 3 Workout B - if you plan to use a heavy or thick powerlifting belt (6") in Stage 4, I would suggest going with a light or thin (4") belt in this phase. I would expect this would apply more so to the neural/advanced lifter than the hypertrophy/beginner program option.

I mentioned a number of other tips earlier on in the sections on deadlifting, including :

1. How to select the bar based on the degree of knurling; and
2. Why you should consider training in track pants.

These points both apply here also.

Deadlifts – MG/OB : This is the overload option for the deadlift, providing exposure to supra-maximal loads. To perform this lift, I want you to find blocks to place the weights on. Ideally the starting bar high will be high shin, just under the knees. In the absence of specially designed lifting blocks you could place your plates on 20 kg plates laid flat, or even the support bases for the steps in the Step Classes.

There are fewer risks than with the squat overload option, but the obvious concern is the fact you are going to be lifting heavier. You are looking to use a load that you could not at this stage do a full range deadlift with. It is important you stay in line and 'tight'.

I have allowed up to 2 work sets at this lift but one set will suffice most. If you are going with 2 sets, you have the option of using step loading – going slightly heavier on the second set.

You may feel a little bit awkward at first with this lift as the higher starting position gives a different feel, which is why a few reps for a warm up set may be appropriate. Not that your body needs warm up by this stage – but a technical rehearsal may be invaluable.

Deadlift – MG/OG : This set sees the bar (or at least the weight plates!) back on the ground. As you did in the squat workout at this stage, you are going to go back down in load and do a set with a rep number just above your first work set reps. Again ideally, if your load selection has been smart and you have not induced too much fatigue, you may be able to perform the requested reps at or just below the load you used in the first work set. Now this is despite it being a medium bar position, a potentially weaker squat position.

But don't be discouraged if you cannot maintain the exact load as you did in the first work set. If possible, stay fairly close. But forget ideals - use your technical and strength levels as a guide – you must use a load that allows you to maintain technique within the desired parameters.

Deadlift – SOB : As per the description on this lift provided earlier, this deadlift variation requires you to stand on a block. How high is the block? Based on my guess of most peoples flexibility and technical ability the block may be as low as a 20 kg plate on it's side. I am referring to a plate that is about 1-2" thick. If you are a rare person with better flexibility and technique, go higher. The limitation in height is this – you need to be able to have your feet under the bar in the start!

I cannot stress enough – if you cannot attain the same starting position as per the conventional, off-the-ground deadlift (pelvis in line with trunk, shoulder blades retracted, etc.), don't do it! Only go as high as your individual flexibility and technique allow.

Now raising the body like this reduces the strength potential (the higher you go the more so). So respect this in your load selection, and place the same expectations of avoiding technical breakdown as you would with any exercise in one of my programs. Don't use a load or a height that denies this technique! If you had to choose between the two, I would rather you go high and light than low and heavy (when I am talking about height differences here I am only talking a difference of a few inches maximum).

Forget about the belt here!

Stiff Legged Deadlift - MG/round over : In this version, the movement starts from the top, in a standing position. Hold the bar with a medium grip (grip just outside your legs), bend the knees slightly, but don't allow the knee angle to change during the lift. Now as you flex forward at the waist, you can round over in the spine. Since Angel Spassov and a few other visitors popularized the so-called 'Bulgarian Squat' (a lunge) and the 'Romanian Deadlift' (a stiff legged deadlift) people have felt obliged to use a chest-up/flat back only position on this and similar lifts. Yes, it is OK to round over! We did the chest up one last time. It is more isolated and a rounded back is more integrated – I like to use them all!

Go down as far as you can i.e. as far as your hamstrings and lower back will take you. If you need to you can stand on a block but not many people are really that flexible!

Stage 3– Concluding Comments

I know that many of you, upon first reading this workout, will wonder where the other exercises are! *'Perhaps I accidentally left them out?'*, you may be thinking! Well, I didn't. Just the two exercises per workout is all I had in mind! With the longer rest periods indicated, plan for a workout durations similar to earlier stages however.

And remember – don't try to get super strong in week 1 of this stage – use it as an 'exposure week'. Doing this will give you extra strength in itself into week two, and go hard in the final week!

Stage 4

Stage 4 – Overview

The final stage – the period where those who have played by the rules I have laid out in this book are going to see the rewards! Expect PBs (personal bests) in this phase!

I have reduced the number of exercises and raised the number of sets per exercise. The advantage of this irrespective of which muscle group is that you provide specialization through increased rehearsal and fatigue on lesser muscle groups. The downside is you may lose or detrain in qualities or muscle groups not as highly targeted as before.

Now any downside can be handled in the short term by addressing it in subsequent programs. So any downside experienced in Stage 4 by reducing number of exercises can be addressed in Stage 1 of the next phase by raising the number of exercises. So no big deal, except in some cases handling the psycho-babble in your head such as *'but am I really doing enough different exercises?'*.

If you are following the linear periodization plan you will be going lower in reps and doing less exercises in this stage compared to Stage 3. If you are going to work the alternating plan, you will be using this program after Stage 2.

I also want to make sure you get the loading protocol that dominates this phase right. You will be using a form of step or wave loading, depending on the level of advancement you are working at.   Step loading involves increased load in subsequent work sets, whereas wave loading sees the load alternate up and down as the sets progress. All are then followed by what I call a 'back off' set.

The critical key to load selection in wave loading is to avoid total fatigue from any of the early sets. If you don't respect this you may negate the potential neural 'dis-inhibition' that step and wave loading offer! To assist you I have provided some samples loading patterns for each of the three protocols – see later in this stage.

You may be familiar with my usual emphasis on the concept that load isn't everything, and that technique and recruitment patterns should be stressed first, as a priority. Now if you have done this – or at least I hope that has been the emphasis, particularly in Stage 1 and 2. Now I am going to replace loading as the priority. Not at the expense of technique, but if I am ever going to allow some drift from optimal technique, it will be in this phase. Not a lot of technical breakdown, but it may happen. If technical breakdown does occur, we place special focus in the start of our subsequent four stage program on re-correcting the lift and joint angle at which technical breakdown may occur.

In essence Stage 4 is a maximal strength phase. It is about loading!

The number of exercises per workout is less in this stage – very low in fact – is some cases, just one exercise! Yes, just one exercise. And isn't it great fun when you can put all your effort into just one exercise! Ever wanted to get good at doing the basic movements? Well now's your chance, because with my relatively low volume approach, using only one exercise allows a fairly high number of sets on that exercise (all of them would you believe!). And when you do this you get the chance to rehearse the skill component of the lift. Provided of course you have a skill component in the way you do them! If you are following my guidelines, you will appreciate the need and benefit of developing the skill in the early stages, and getting strong within that skill or movement pattern as the program progress.

Ever wondered how the powerlifters get that 'thick' look? My perspective on this is that one contributor is regular exposure to high load, the other is high volume of sets on less exercise. And this program gives both. You don't want to be a powerlifter? Irrespective of your end goals, your physique will benefit from training like one from time to time!

What about muscle balance? Well provided we addressed this earlier in the program, we can throw caution to the wind and focus on a more narrow approach for this stage. Of course, when you start your next program, you will go back and address the potential imbalances that this stage may have produced by again prioritizing the weaker, neglected muscle groups....

There is a skill and strategy to succeeding with low rep/high load sets. In brief, if you enter the set with a low level of arousal, you will lift little, and get little benefit. In low rep/high load sets, the window of opportunity is very brief and you need to take a whole new perspective into the workout to optimize the outcome. You will benefit from using focus and arousal methods to optimize your load capacity.

Now what's in store in Stage 4?

With the **abdominal program** in this stage, if there were ever a stage that you would more likely put the abs at the end of the program, it would be Stage 3 and Stage 4. However please be prepared to make this decision as fits your situation now! If your abs are still lagging or if you are enjoying/appreciating the benefits of placing them first, don't feel bad about retaining them first in the workout. At the same time, placing them back to the end of the workout in Stage 4, knowing that in your next program you can bring them back up to first in the sequence for a while, is quite acceptable! My main concern is that you don't fatigue neurally in a maximal strength phase by placing them first.

The **upper body program** in this stage dominates over the lower body program. Within the upper body program, the upper body pushing (horizontal and vertical) dominates over pulling. This is so because the first exercise on the first workout of the week is bench press. Due to the low number of exercises, this is a fantastic opportunity to specialize on the bench press and chin up!

In the **lower body** training, you are going to continue the quad dominant approach from phase 3 i.e. quad dominant exercises will occur first in the training week. Irrespective of whether you are following the linear periodization plan or the alternating periodization plan, you will be going lower in reps. Again, you have an excellent opportunity to specialize in the squat and deadlift!

The following provides **general information about this stage of the program**:

This program is based on standard setting. Do a set, take the (long) rest indicated or thereabouts. Do the next set. Etc. After all, other than bench or bench (A day) or chin and chin (C day), there isn't much else to do other than check out the scenario. Note take shorter rest periods on the warm up sets.

One thing that usually happens when you take up an exercise station for 40 minutes or so (i.e. 5 sets of 5 mins rest + work set time etc) is that you will get people either wanting to take over that piece of equipment (if they are the rude type) or people asking *"have you finished yet?"* (No, I just loaded the bar up to 300 kgs as an exercise in art!). I don't recommend you sit on or too close to the work stations – makes it harder for the conscious and subconscious mind to increase arousal levels when you come into the vicinity of the work station for the set if you have just been relaxing on it – which leaves a situation of 'how do I guard and keep my work station?

Some place a towel or similar on the work station. Even if you do this you will want to sit a few meters from the work station where you can see it, so you can discourage others from stripping the bar. Of course you are happy to 'work in' with someone, provided they have the bar loaded back up to where you had it when you want it.

Should you use spotters? DEFINITELY. A trained competent spotter required. If you have any doubts about them, have them work with you in your last warm up set as a dress rehearsal. Remember, my definition of a spotter is someone to be there so you don't have to lose focus wondering what might happen IF you cannot finish the rep. Don't pick weights knowing you have a spotter. Lift the weights with peace of mind your safety is taken care of should the unthinkable happen – but don't select and use loads with the intent of giving your spotter an upright row workout! And make sure they understand what speed to lift the bar should you fail in the concentric phase – my preference is for the bar to be lifted at the same speed as the average concentric speed for that set. Any slower and you will be inducing too much fatigue.

To assist you with loading decisions in this stage, I have provided the following guidelines – see the below for generalized guidelines on what type of jumps may be involved in the step and wave loading.

Now go and *Get Buffed!* ™

Hypertrophy/Lower Training Age Option

Sample loading pattern in week 1 for the 4x4 step load method (hypertrophy/lower training age)

Warm up sets
1 x 20kgs @ 10 reps
1 x 40kgs @ 8 reps
1 x 60kgs @6 reps

Work sets
1 x 80kgs @ 4 reps
1 x 82.5 kgs @ 4 reps
1 x 85 kgs @ 4 reps
1 x 87.5 kgs @ 4 reps
1 x 60kgs @ 8-10 reps
1 x 40 kgs @ 15-20 reps

An example of weekly progressions is given below :

	Wk 1	Wk 2	Wk 3
WU x 10	20	20	20
WU x 8	40	42.5	45
WU x 6	60	62.5	65
Work x 4	80.0	82.5	85.0
Work x 4	82.5	85.0	87.5
Work x 4	85.0	87.5	90.0
Work x 4	87.5	90.0	92.5
Work x 8-10	60	60 or 62.5	60 or 62.5 or 65
Work x 15-20	40	40 or 42.5	40 or 42.5 or 45

Hypertrophy-neural/Intermediate Training Age Option

Sample loading pattern in week 1 for the 4x3 wave load method (hypertrophy-neural/intermediate training age)

Warm up sets
1x20kgs @ 10 reps
1 x 40kgs @ 8 reps
1 x 60kgs @5 reps
1x80kgs @ 3 reps (optional)

Work sets
1 x 100kgs @ 3 reps
1 x 105.0 kgs @ 3 reps
1 x 102.5 kgs @ 3 reps
1 x 107.5 kgs @ 3 reps
1 x 80kgs @ 8-10 reps
1 x 60 kgs @ 10-15 reps

An example of weekly progressions is given below :

	Wk 1	Wk 2	Wk 3
WU x 10	20	20	20
WU x 8	40	42.5	45
WU x 5	60	62.5	65
WU x 3	80	82.5	85
Work x 3	100.0	102.5	105.0
Work x 3	105.0	107.5	110.0
Work x 3	102.5	105.0	107.5
Work x 3	107.5	110.0	112.5
Work x 8-10	80	80 or 82.5	80 or 82.5 or 85
Work x 10-15	60	60 or 62.5	60 or 62.5 or 65

Neural/Advanced Training Age Option

Sample loading pattern in week 1 for the 5x2 wave load method (neural/advanced training age)

Warm up sets
1x20kgs @ 10 reps
1 x 50kgs @ 6 reps
1 x 80kgs @4 reps
1x100kgs @ 2 reps (optional)

Work sets
1 x 120kgs @ 2 reps
1 x 130 kgs @ 2 reps
1 x 125 kgs @ 2 reps
1 x 135 kgs @ 2 reps
1 x 130 kgs @ 2 reps (optional set)
1 x 100kgs @ 5-8 reps
1 x 80 kgs @ 8-12 reps

An example of weekly progressions is given below :

	Wk 1	Wk 2	Wk 3
WU x 10	20	25	30
WU x 6	50	55	60
WU x 4	80	85	90
WU x 2	100	105	110
Work x 2	120	125	130
Work x 2	130	135	140
Work x 2	125	130	135
Work x 2	135	140	145
Work x 2 (option)	130	135	140
Work x 5-8	100	100 or 105	100 or 105 or 110
Work x 8-12	80	80 or 85	80 or 85 or 90

Stage 4 – Warm Up / Stretching / Abdominal / Control Drills

A & C Day

Exercise	Warm up	Work	Speed	Rest
Warm Up	optional 5-15 minutes of light aerobic type activity e.g. stationary bike			
Stretch	10-20 minutes of upper body stretching			
Abdominals				
Knee up ball	nil	1-2x10-20	201	2m
Partner leg throws	15 at easy	1x5-15 With ext load	*	2m
Full V-sits	nil	1-2x5-15	10*	2m
Control Drills				
Flutters	nil	1x10-15	202	0-30s
Scarecrow	nil	1x 10	202	0-30s
Side Lying Ext DB Rotation	nil	1x10	202	0-30s
Prone Limited Range DB Row	nil	1x10	202	0-30s
Workout				

Stage 4 : A & C Day – Abdominal Exercise Descriptions

Here are descriptions of the abdominal exercises involved in A and C day, Stage 4 of the *Get Buffed!* ™ II (Get More Buffed!) four (4) stage program.

Knee Up on ball : You could move on to this no matter which level you got to last program, unless of course you find this movement just too difficult (or if you don't have access to a SWIS ball – in either case, work on progression from where you were in the last stage of this program).

Now this exercise will involve a SWIS ball (or whatever you want to call it – you will see it called various names in different countries).

Place the ball in front of a prone bench. Ideally the ball height will be similar to the bench height. If not look for a different size ball or different height bench! Now place both knees on the ball and both hands on the bench. You will in a kneeling position.

Keeping your hands (palms) parallel on the bench, arms straight, extend the knees backwards until the body is almost straight from the shoulder to the knees (the body won't be parallel to the ground, but can and should in the ideal end position, form a straight line between the knee and the shoulders.

Two things here. Firstly, you may find the need to adjust the knees on the ball in the start position, so that in the end position you are not rolling off the ball. If you find yourself rolling off the ball (in the sagital plane or the long axis of the body, not sideways off!), don't panic, just experiment with you knee position in the start position till you get it right!

The other point I want to discuss is the end point. Is everyone going to be able to straighten out the knees to this point and be able to recover? No. Give it a go. Worse case, you fall on the floor. Ideally the floor is not too far away! But if you cannot recover from the position and continue to rep at least a minimum of 5 reps, don't extend out as far. In subsequent workouts look to improve the range you use or the reps you do or both.

If you are very advanced you can look to extend the arms out further. This will require some upper body strength also (as will the base movement), as again, despite what the some suggest, Swiss ball exercises are rarely if ever isolated movements!

Don't feel the need to go fast with this movement. Take it slow, get the range, and build on the reps!

Do I have any fine tips like how to hold your hips? No, as I discussed earlier, my training philosophy is to drill the movement in the early days in a manner that you do without thinking the technique you want, at least generally speaking. This low level coaching/personal training technique of giving you 100 tips to think about when doing a high level movement, most of which are impossible or irrelevant, is not the approach I recommend!

Are there any back issues with this movement? Remember what I say – the only one who will be able to make that judgment is you – if it hurts or you suspect if may cause harm, don't do it! Also note that I recommend you go to a straight body position (straight line from shoulders to knees), not a saggy back position! This could increase lower back stresses, and there is no need to go there!

Notes :

Speed of movement – Controlled movement at 201 or 301.

Selecting appropriate level - Start conservatively in your range, and progress over the subsequent workouts and weeks in range and reps; ensure that no lower back (lumbar) pain is being experienced.

Partner Leg Throws : Lie on the ground and get someone to stand over your head, their feet either side of your ears. Grab hold of their ankles with each hand.

This is a dynamic, high stress movement so if you have lower back issues, look for an alternative straight away!

Have your partner grab your ankles as a result of you lifting your legs up to them. Keep your legs together throughout this exercise. Now have your partner throw your legs to the ground. In the first set (the warm up set) have them throw or push them down gently and only in a straight line. In the work set, get them to progressively increase the amount of force they push with, and vary the angle they throw your legs down at.

Your goal is to resist the movement before the legs touch the ground and get your legs back up to the partner as fast as you can. This is a great movement when you get into the higher levels of force and greater angle variations, where you can have your legs thrown almost 90 degrees to the long axis of your trunk.

A tip to remember – have the partner grab your legs and pause after each rep. If they don't you tend to anticipate the movement and use elastic energy. It's much harder work if they pause in the holding of your legs before throwing them. Also, have your partner use basically a chest pass technique. Let them know that provided you are up to it, by the end the of work set/s, they can or may be using their full force in the throw!

Another tip for the person throwing – have them vary the angle, be balanced in how many they do to each side, and try to avoid them being able to anticipate where the next leg throw is going!

Notes :

Speed of movement - This is a dynamic movement, indicated by the symbol '*'. Go both down and up as fast as you can, but no touching feet on ground! Your goal should be to minimize the amount of range that results from the partners push.

Selecting appropriate level – Have the partner start conservatively in their throws, both in force as well as angle variation.

Full V-sits : You had better done the ground work in the lead up to this variation! Lie on your back on the ground with your arms out over your head, parallel and resting on the ground, and your legs out straight also. Just like a diver reaching up to the sky only you are on your back on the ground.

Now pivoting from the waist, raise (flex) your legs and arms simultaneously, keeping both legs and arms straight, and have them meet (ideally) at the top i.e. where the legs and arms are equal distance or angle from the ground. It is a lazy option to meet one side or the other of the vertical line. For example if your trunk flexion was weak but your hip flexion strong, you might be tempted to meet the legs and arms closer to the head side of vertical. If your trunk flexion was strong and your hip flexion weak, you may be tempted to meet the legs and arms on the feet side of the vertical. Do the hard yards – have them meet in the vertical position!

Don't be surprised if this takes a bit of practice and co-ordination, and don't expect to do too many reps, at least not initially!

I find this movement less stressful on the lower back than the modified v-sit from the previous stage, but that will depend on how you execute the movement. If you are doing it in the way I describe the pelvis will round with the body (hip should posteriorly rotate). But if you lift the legs ahead of lifting the arms, for example, you could strain your lower back with the anterior rotation of the pelvis.

Do I give any specific cues? No more than the information above. I keep it simple – the arms and legs leave the ground simultaneously and meet in the vertical position – simple!

Do you need external load? Not many will! But if you did you would be looking for ankle weights and holding a weight in the arms. Don't get delusional – get it right before even contemplating this!

Notes :

Speed of movement – Explosive movement at 10*. Lift as fast as your strength and coordination allow, and lower under some control but no need for slow.

Selecting appropriate level – There is pretty much only one level in this variation! If you find it too much (physically, not co-ordination – if it is coordination just keep practicing!) then return to lower level variations!

Stage 4 – Warm Up / Stretching / Abdominal / Control Drills

B & D Day

Exercise	Warm up	Work	Speed	Rest
Warm Up	10-20 minutes of light aerobic type activity e.g. stationary bike			
Stretch	20-40 minutes of lower body stretching			
Abdominals				
Partner resisted sit-ups	10 at b/wgt	1x10-20	303	2m
Full range curl ups	15 at b/wgt*	1x10-15	301	2m
Med Ball sit ups	1x15-25 with a light ball	1x15-25 heavier ball	10*	2m
Control Drills				
Light leg extensions	nil	1x10-15	202	0-30s
Prone lying single leg hip / thigh extensions	nil	1x10	202	0-30s
Side Lying Lateral Leg Raise	nil	1x10	202	0-30s
Co-Contraction Lunge	nil	1x10	202	0-30s
Lying Supine Single Leg Hip/Thigh Extension	nil	1x5-10	202	0-30s
Assisted Squat	nil	1x10	202	0-30s
Workout				

* only need to do a warm up set if you plan to use external resistance in the work sets. If you don't plan to use external resistance in the work sets, ignore warm up set.

Get Buffed!™ II

Stage 4 : B & D Day – Abdominal Exercise Descriptions

Here are descriptions of the abdominal exercises involved in B and D day, Stage 4 of the *Get Buffed!* ™ II (Get More Buffed!) four (4) stage program.

Partner Resisted Sit-up : You are going to need a partner again. Make sure they are switched on and listen to you. A sadistic partner here could make things very tough! This is the same body position that I have had you use throughout in the curl up - lying on your back on the ground, knees bent to about 90 degrees, and feet flat on the floor. Your feet are not to be anchored under anything. Then you sit up or curl up the trunk, ideally to a full sitting position.

The only difference now is that you are going to have the partner apply light resistance to your chest during the setup, and again against your chest during the lowering. I stress here – light resistance. You will not need much resistance to give you the outcome I am chasing. For example, you don't want your setup speed to be much slower than it would be with a weight on your chest. You will find that with excessive partner force you will either be too slow in the lift or you may not be able to sit up at all.

You may also require the partner to reduce the force during the set as you fatigue. So you need a smart partner who understands what you are trying to achieve

Now in the lower part of the exercise, you may think you can handle more force applied by the partner, and this may be the case – but believe me, it's a lot less force than you may think! Your lowering should be smooth and constant, not collapsing at any stage. So also have the partner receptive to your force curve – i.e. the fact that your strength changes as you go through the joint angles. As you hit a weaker joint angle, you want them to back off on the force. You want to maintain a constant lowering speed, taking about 2-3 seconds to complete the lowering.

So don't turn the lift into an arm wrestle!

Notes :

Speed of movement – Attempt to accelerate up, realizing that the force applied by the partner will cause the movement to appear slow. No pause needed. Control the lowering, aiming for a constant speed, no collapsing.

Arm positions – Pretty irrelevant – probably best to keep the arms parallel to the ground rather than across the body if you want the chest free for force to be applied by the partner.

Selecting appropriate level - The only way to really know what level of force from the partner is appropriate is to have the partner experiment during the first few reps. If in doubt, get them to push less.

Full Range Curls Ups : Option within this exercise include the use of a Swiss ball, or a prone bench.

Lie on you back with the upper back across a Swiss ball or a prone bench. If you are using a prone bench, your body will be perpendicular (right angles) to the bench. The advantage of the ball is more comfort and support, but both (bench and ball) are options.

You are probably going to need to have your feet anchored, but this is not a necessity. If you want to reduce the hip flexor involvement or if you don't have a partner or way of hooking or anchoring the feet, no problem – as long as you don't fall off the device you are using, and provided you are not compromising your range because of this.

Now, with your arms across your chest (or higher on the head if you want more resistance), allow your upper body to extend as far as it can. In most cases, unless you have physical weakness or other limitation, it will until your head is nearly on the ground – then sit back up from there.

If you did need to add resistance (and I don' think this will apply to many!), you can hold weight on your chest but don't assume this until you do the required reps at bodyweight!

Notes :

Speed of movement – Perform this movement with control during the lowering, and then control again on the way up. No pause needed.

Arm positions – Start with arms crossed over the chest. The placement of the hands will alter the level of difficulty. The further the hands are above the head, the harder the movement.

Selecting appropriate level – Don't rush into external load – see if you get the reps with bodyweight first, with your arms crossed on your chest. If you then feel you need more load, take the hands to touching the head, and then above the head, before moving to external load. With external load, on the chest is the most comfortable option but holding it at head level or above will increase the resistance.

Med Ball Sit-ups : This is a great exercise if you enjoy catching and passing. If not, look for an alternative! You are going to need a medicine ball (preferably a range of medicine balls e.g. 1 kg through to 5 kg) and a partner.

One of you lie on the ground with your needs bent, then sit up. The other stands in front of the lying person, with the med ball. How far in front? How far do you want to throw and catch? Basically, the further apart you are from the thrower, potentially the greater the work you will do. Start off by standing about a meter away from the feet of the lying person.

The standing person throws the ball at the lying person, who is seated with their arms out in anticipation. More like drops it on them initially – the hard throwing is never really needed. The lying person catches the ball, takes it over their head as they lower back down, and has the ball touch the ground above their head at the same time they are lying flat down on the ground. They immediately sit up and bring the ball up with them, throwing the ball as they reach the top of the sit up. There is a variation where you can throw the ball as you sit up but that's more difficult.

Now as the person on the ground warms up to the movement, the thrower can do a few things to make it harder, more challenging, and basically more fun. These include :

1. Use a heavier ball (usually use a lighter one in the warm up sets, a heavier one in the work sets). How heavy? Depends on how fast or slow you believe the movement should be conducted. If you wanted to specifically rehearse explosiveness, don't go so heavier that the speed of the sit up is compromised too much!

2. Throw the ball harder. You don't need a heavier ball in this case, but you need a reason to do this. For example, you are increasing the forces in the eccentric phase more than the concentric phases, so you need a rationale for this.

3. Throw the ball in varying directions. All in places that can be caught, but instead of straight at the chest/arms, try throwing off to the side, or a bit higher above their head. Remember for every throw off-center to the right, do one to the left. Again, apart from the fun, you need a reason. One could be that you are working a greater variety of trunk muscles in doing this and this is a very valid reason! Another may be that the person on the ground will benefit from being challenged in the reaction and catching skills. I find this to be great for example with basketball players. Make sure that you are realistic – that all things being equal they will catch the ball!

Now there is an option where you both get down on the ground and work together, or at least taking reps in turn. This is more time efficient and a great option.

Notes :

Speed of movement – Go down and up as fast as you can.

Selecting appropriate level - Start with a lighter ball, and an easier throw. As the person gets warmer, and as their abilities improve, increase the weight of ball, how hard you throw it, and or the direction you throw the ball in.

Arm positions - Not relevant.

Stage 4, Option 1 - Hypertrophy / Lower Training Age

A Day

Exercise	Warm up	Work	Speed	Rest
Bench Press (MG/LB/FD/Arch)	10/8/6	4x4	211	4m
		1x8-10	211	
		1x15-20	211	

NB Step load the 4x4 work sets

Stage 4, Option 2 - Hypertrophy-neural / Intermediate Training Age

A Day

Exercise	Warm up	Work	Speed	Rest
Bench Press (MG/LB/FD/Arch)	10/8/5 opt 1x3	4x3	211	4-5m
		1x8-10	211	
		1x10-15	211	

NB Wave load the 4x3 work sets

Stage 4, Option 3 - Neural/Advanced Training Age

A Day

Exercise	Warm up	Work	Speed	Rest
Bench Press	10/6/4	5x2	211	5-6m
(MG/LB/FD/Arch)	opt 1x2	1x5-8	211	
		1x8-12	211	

NB Wave load the 5x2 work sets

Stage 4 : A Day - Exercise Descriptions

Here are descriptions of the exercises involved in A day, Stage 4 of the *Get Buffed!* ™ II (Get More Buffed!) four (4) stage program.

Bench Press : (medium grip, low bar, feet down, medium arch) Take a medium grip on the bench press. For most this will be with the little fingers inside the lines on the Olympic bar. You will lower the bar down to the lower portion of the chest - this is a strong position, allowing a greater arc in the bar movement and greater lat involvement. Your feet are to be on the ground.

I want you to arch as much as you can. There are many ways to get into an arch, but the outcome is the same. The hips and head are in contact with the bench, but as close to each other as you can contort them to be! Your feet are flat on the ground, slightly turned out, and your knees are at an acute degree of flexion. Take some tension and load through your legs and buttocks. Remember the greater the arch, potentially the heavier the loads you can lift – so get it organized! You may want to do some passive hyperextension prone on the ground prior to the bench to warm up this position, and after each set I like to do some cradle position on the bench before getting up to reverse the hyper-extended position.

I encourage you to familiarize yourself with the tips regarding benching as the load is increased that I shared with you in Stage 3 of this program.

Stage 4, Option 1 - Hypertrophy / Lower Training Age

B Day

Exercise	Warm up	Work	Speed	Rest
Squat (LB/M-WS)	1x10/1x8/ 1x6/ opt 1x4	4x4 1x10-12 1x15-20	201	4-5m

NB. Step load the 4 x 4 work sets.

Stage 4, Option 2 - Hypertrophy-neural / Intermediate Training Age

B Day

Exercise	Warm up	Work	Speed	Rest
Squat (LB/M-WS)	1x10/1x8/ 1x5/ opt 1x3	4x3 1x6-8 1x10-15	201	5-6m

NB. wave load the 4 x 3 work sets.

Stage 4, Option 3 - Neural/Advanced Training Age

B Day

Exercise	Warm up	Work	Speed	Rest
Squat (LB/M-WS)	1x10/1x8/ 1x5/ opt 1x3	4x2 1x4-6 1x8-12	201	6-7m

NB. wave load the 4 x 2 work sets.

Stage 4 : B Day - Exercise Descriptions

Here are descriptions of the exercises involved in B day, Stage 4 of the *Get Buffed!* ™ II (Get More Buffed!) four (4) stage program.

Squat – LB/M-WS : With the bar on a squat rack, approach the bar and place the bar on a low bar height on the shoulders behind the head. What is low bar? Any lower and it would fall off is one way of describing it! Another is to say a bit lower than last stage (e.g. ½ to 1"). Another way is to teach you how to identify 3 different practical and safe heights for the bar on your upper back – I trust you used the highest position in Stage 1, the medium position in Stage 2, and now we are going to use all three in this stage!

When you step backwards out of the racks assume a medium to wide stance (shoulder width or just outside). I prefer a shoulder width stance for running sport athletes and those concerned with hypertrophy of the legs, but those pursuing loading only may take a wider stance if they wish. Make sure you confirm your stance in the warm up sets and don't do it any differently during the work sets!

Confirm your technique as per my recommendations.

As the load is being raised even more, the issues of wearing a belt and or knee wraps will no doubt arise. If you plan to compete in squatting or deadlifting, now may be the time to use all the powerlifting apparatus you are allowed to wear in competition. If you used a 4" belt in Stage 3, consider the 6" belt in Stage 4. If you didn't wear a belt in Stage 3, only consider the 4" belt now.

And the same applies to knee wraps – if you plan to compete in squatting or deadlifting, now may be the time to use all the powerlifting apparatus you are allowed to wear in competition in this phase. As with the belt, this should be more of a consideration for the neural/advanced lifter than the hypertrophy/beginner program option.

I want to make it clear that neither belts nor knee wraps are required, but they are options.

Stage 4, Option 1 - Hypertrophy / Lower Training Age

C Day

Exercise	Warm up	Work	Speed	Rest
Chin Up (neutral medium grip)	10/8/6	4x4 1x8-10 1x15-20	211 211 211	4m

NB Step load the 4x4 work sets.

Stage 4, Option 2 - Hypertrophy-neural / Intermediate Training Age

C Day

Exercise	Warm up	Work	Speed	Rest
Chin up (neutral medium grip) opt 1x3	10/8/5	4x3 1x8-10 1x10-15	211 211 211	4-5m

NB Wave load the 4x3 work sets.

Stage 4, Option 3 - Neural/Advanced Training Age

C Day

Exercise	Warm up	Work	Speed	Rest
Chin up	10/6/4	5x2	211	5-6m
(neutral medium grip) opt 1x2		1x5-8	211	
		1x8-12	211	

NB Wave load the 5x2 work sets.

Stage 4 : C Day - Exercise Descriptions

Here are descriptions of the exercises involved in C day, Stage 4 of the *Get Buffed!* ™ II (Get More Buffed!) four (4) stage program.

Chin Up : (neutral/medium grip, i.e. palms facing towards each other, shoulder width). Take a shoulder width grip with palms facing towards each other. If your gym doesn't have this option, don't panic. Use whatever you find to be your strongest grip position. Allow the feet to come off the ground slowly, without inducing any body sway. Cross the feet at the ankle and tuck them up behind you. Pull straight up and finish the pull with the chin over the handgrip level. Don't do another rep if this pulling range is not met.

Avoid swaying in the chin up using the techniques I recommended earlier. This sway can be made worse by the external load or the way you are attaching it to your body, and there will be a lot of external load sets in this program. I like the old 'rope and belt' method, and I clamp the external load (usually a weight plate) between my upper thighs. This keeps the load still and central.

If you want a visual display/discussion about how I want the chin ups done, check out the *Get Buffed!*™ *Video Series*, which covers all the exercises from the original *Get Buffed!*™ book (for end users, available at www.getbuffed.net), or the *How To Teach Strength Training Video Series* (available at www.kingports.net).

I also encourage you to familiarize yourself with the tips about chin ups that I shared with you in Stage 3 of this program series.

I also made the point in Stage 3 that if you cannot get the reps in the final back off set (or both of the back off sets) at bodyweight, use the lat pulldown instead. Or use the lat pulldown in a superset to compliment the reps if you don't hit the target on the chin bar. Either way, show speed in the lift!

Stage 4, Option 1 - Hypertrophy / Lower Training Age

D Day

Exercise	Warm up	Work	Speed	Rest
Deadlift (Alt. Grip)	1x10/1x8/ 1x6/opt 1x4	4x4 1x10-12 1x15-20	201	4-5m

NB Step load the 4x4 work sets.

Stage 4, Option 2 - Hypertrophy-neural / Intermediate Training Age

D Day

Exercise	Warm up	Work	Speed	Rest
Deadlift (Alt. Grip)	1x10/1x8/ 1x5/opt 1x3	4x3 1x6-8 1x10-15	201	5-6m

NB Wave load the 4x3 work sets.

Stage 4, Option 3 - Neural/Advanced Training Age

D Day

Exercise	Warm up	Work	Speed	Rest
Deadlift (Alt. Grip)	1x10/1x8/ 1x5/opt 1x3	4x2 1x4-6 1x8-12	201	6-7m

NB Wave load the 4x2 work sets.

Stage 4 : D Day - Exercise Descriptions

Here are descriptions of the exercises involved in D day, Stage 4 of the *Get Buffed!* ™ II (Get More Buffed!) four (4) stage program.

Deadlifts – MG/OG : Using a medium (just outside your legs), reverse grip (i.e. palms facing each other), and starting from the bottom position, weight rested on the ground. It is critical you confirm your technique as per my recommendations earlier in this program.

Note I want you to reverse grip in this phase. If you are unsure which hand should face forward and which hand should face backwards, experiment until comfortable. But I strongly recommend you do not change over during the work sets. Stay with the combination you used in the warm up sets. There is injury potential in not respecting this suggestion.

The use of chalk to increase grip retention is critical. I would only recommend wrist straps (that anchor your grip to the bar) as a last option.

I have addressed the use a belt in relation to deadlifting previously.

Stage 4 – Concluding Comments

So here is your opportunity to develop that big bench press, squat, chin up and deadlift! Be smart about it, avoiding over-training and injury. Learn to master focus, imagery, and arousal during this time, to exploit the window of opportunity. Note whatever technical breakdown may have occurred to be addressed in later phases. And in your next program after this one, counter the imbalances that may have arisen during this stage of narrow focus in regards to exercise selection.

If you have had the discipline and belief to stick with my recommendations for the full four stages, I trust it has been a rewarding and educational experience! Thanks for participating!

Throughout this book (and the whole *Get Buffed!*™ series) I have aimed to educate you on the topic of training so that you could apply this knowledge now and in future to a more individualized program (and perhaps even guide your coach or trainer to this end result!).

In conclusion, I trust that your diligent involvement produces a combination of both short term (physical) and long term (knowledge) changes that have a positive impact on your life!

Chapter 12
Fools Gold
Helping you resist the temptations!

Before finishing this book I want to ensure I have left you with my suggestions for avoiding some of the training temptations present in strength training, and the strength training environment. I believe the following techniques are the fools gold of weight training :

- ❑ Cheat movements
- ❑ Movements using momentum
- ❑ Limited range movements

I am not saying don't do them. Rather, don't base your training on these methods. If you do, I believe you will not achieve what you could achieve.

Many may claim that these methods dominate in their training because of the Achilles heel of conventional non-cheat movements using constant external load (e.g. barbell) - that you are only over-loading the weakest joint angles in the force curve. That is, the weight you use is determined by what the weakest part of the movement will allow, and therefore you don't get to overload the stronger joint angles. And the claim is made that these methods overcome this limitation.

This may be true, but to use these methods for the majority of time is like throwing out the baby with the bathwater. Non-cheat movements may be flawed in perfection, but what's the benefit of dominating in training with more flawed methods?!

You might wonder now why I am taking such a stance against the most universally popular strength training methods! Let's face it – the popularity of these methods has nothing to do with their medium or long-term efficacy! Their popularity is based on the immediate gratification. Gratification based on the perception a person gives when using these techniques! 'Hey, check me out! Aren't I strong!' Get over it!

If you base your load selection on what it takes to impress a transient group of relative strangers who may observe you for fractions of a second – you need to take a reality check. They may go home with a short term memory equivalent to *'Gee, that guy in the red tank top was strong because he had x on the bar!'* You, on the other hand, go home and wake up the next day and the next day and the next day (you get my point!) with the outcome of your decisions. So don't make emotional decisions based on impressing others when it comes to a long-term goal! Get rid the habit of feeling the need to impress others as the basis for your training decisions!

Never assume that the load a person is bouncing around like a circus act is indicative of how big and strong they are. What makes it worse, so many pursuing hypertrophy go down this 'see how strong I am because I am lifting so much weight' path! In fact, conventional movements (i.e. non-cheat) as your training base (i.e. dominant method) may be more effective for hypertrophy anyway! And if you are truly a strength athlete (which amongst the total population of the strength gyms around the world would be less than 1%!), then chances are the specificity of the pauses or the velocities in your sport will dictate the appropriate average velocity and pauses in your training! Not some circus trick aimed at creating a fleeting impression on a stranger!

So that's the primary reason I believe these methods are so popular – they allow short term emotional gratification in those whose focus is more about impressing others with smoke and mirrors than the long term training effect.

The second reason I believe they are so popular is because of market research. Someone sees others doing it, assumes it's the way to go, and they do it. The sheep following the sheep! It must be *'the way you do it!'*. I even saw Will on the US day-time soap opera *'Days of our Lives'* doing seated lateral DB raises – and he, yes, you guessed...was using a cheat technique! You fool Will! But I know there will be millions rushing out to copy him! In the same way he or the show producers copied someone else in the gym!

What I am going to do now is spend a moment defining each of these movements, and sharing with you what I like and don't like about them.

Cheat Movements

Definition : I call any movement that uses a joint or muscle that are not the targets of your training to be a cheat movement. If I see a joint movement other than the joint around which the target muscles are – then it's a cheat movement.

Disadvantages of this technique : My initial concern is that you fail to overload the muscle through the full range with this technique. Yes, I know, you are doing them to overload the stronger joint angles. Fine. But what about the weaker joint angles?

Following on from that, my concern (an ever greater concern!) surrounds controlling the variable of cheating. So you just cheated a bit with 100 lbs. At 110 lbs and getting the same reps, did you actually do more work? Were you truly stronger? Or did you just cheat more?

What I see is as the loads are lifted, the person cheats more. And this totally undermines the basis of training – progressive overload!

There is also the concern of increased injury risk with this technique but I believe this has been over-done. If you get conditioned to them, the risks reduce. I have seen track and field throwers doing ballistic movements in the gym with weights that I am sure would tear most of us in two! But they seemed pretty comfortable with it!

Advantages : The first advantage is you can impress others at the time, but I am not even going to respect that with further discussion. On a more valid note, yes, you can use cheat movements to ensure overload on stronger joint angles. And as I have often said, it has more application to pulling movements than pushing movements. Further, when you are in a program or a phase when completing the movement is more important than how you completed it, cheating is a great option. In fact, some base their training on the concept that 'if it moved, it was a rep'!

Movements Using Momentum

Definition : I call these movements any exercise that uses momentum beyond that which is advantageous to the goal.

I am talking about for example bench pressing so far and fast down that your rib cage is compressed and provides upward momentum. Now I know that in the experienced hands of say an elite powerlifter, this technique is used effectively and relatively safely. But I am talking about the average person in the gym, who appears to be determining the breaking strain levels of their rib cage!

I am also talking about using a speed of movement in the eccentric phase that is aimed to reduce the work required to complete the concentric phase. I am talking about the use or absence of pauses between eccentric and concentric contractions. What I am getting into is the use of elastic energy and that is a whole new ball game. You see, you can manipulate elastic energy to reduce or increase muscle work and force created. Put simply, if your goal is to lift as much as you can, you (generally speaking) look to exploit the elastic energy. On the other hand if your goal is to make the muscles work as hard as they can you look to negate the elastic energy.

How do you 'exploit' elastic energy? You lower the weight fast, use a short a range of movement as you can, you don't pause, and you lift as fast as you can. How do you 'negate' elastic energy? You lower slowly, you pause long, and you lift slowly.

When do you want to exploit or negate elastic energy? Again, generally speaking, if your primary concern was how hard the muscles worked, you negate elastic energy. This would be the more appropriate of the two options for hypertrophy training. If your primary concern were how much load you lifted or how fast you lifted it, you would (generally speaking) exploit elastic energy. This would apply to say athletes training in specific strength periods, if the exercises were based on the concept of speed-specificity, at least.

So to finally get to the point – if your goal is to develop muscle size and strength, and you predominantly exploited the elastic energy in your strength training – I would call this using momentum beyond that which is advantageous to the goal! Conversely, if you were a power athlete and your strength training was based around intentionally slow speed movements, I would be concerned for you!

Disadvantages of this technique : The main disadvantage is when the training outcome is different to the training goal. When the bodybuilder uses momentum excessively, or when the power athlete uses controlled movements excessively. And of course, when during the bench press the rib cage cracks and pierces the lungs….Or when the bounce off the chest in the bench press is such that the lifter loses control during the concentric phase and the forehead is threatened (and I have seen this happen)!

Advantages : Appropriate use of momentum manipulation has much to offer. Quite simply, if you want a result, you need to consider some specificity in training. Inappropriate use has nothing to offer. That's the difference. And realistically and in fairness the average weight trainee would have no clue either way! In fact, most people receiving payment to advice and supervise training would probably be found out in this area also.

Limited range movements

Definition : I describe a limited range movement as any movement that is executed in a shorter range than the full range movement that is available for that movement.

So here's another way of looking at it – a range shorter than the normal range for that movement. For example a bench press is normally conducted from full extension to where the bar touches the chest.

Disadvantages of this technique : Again, similar to cheating movements, my initial concern is that all angles aren't trained. In actual fact, if you used limited range exclusively, you ability to use further range may be reduced even in general lift activities. You run the risk of adhesions preventing full range! Now that may be extreme, but let me assure you, a muscle not moved through it's full range during the majority of its use runs the risk of this!

So you are left with no strength development in certain joint angles (often vital ones at that) and you run the risk of reducing range long-term. Reduction of range may result in inhibited function (less power output), more joint friction (accelerated arthritis) and increased nerve related referred pain. That's a lot of disadvantages!

As with the cheating discussion, it also raises the question – did you get stronger? Did you do more work? Or did you just do less range?

For me, set the range, and it doesn't change. If you can't get the range, don't do the rep.

Advantages : Limited range movements probably have more validity and application than the other two movements. When you want to isolate and strength a specific joint angle (isometric) or angles (limited range movement) this is a totally valid option. For example, a competitive powerlifter may be working on their bench lockout. An injured person may be working in a pain free range.

But realistically, of all the people aimlessly displacing molded steel on any given day, I believe less that 1% could justify objectively the use of limited range movements.

In **summary** I have outlined my concerns and the benefits of each of the methods that I called the 'Fools Gold' of weight training. I also said at the outset that the use of these methods was not the problem. The problems occur when they dominated your training. I am not saying that these training options are bad or should never be used. I say clearly that they should make up the minority of your training, not the majority. Specifically, what constitutes minority? I don't have that answer. It's time to get back to the roots of the training process – the answer lies in the individual, and can only be read by those prepared to master the analysis of their own or others training. But to help you out, especially if you are a beginner or beginner-intermediate : there is little call for these methods in the early years of your training!

Conclusion

By now I trust you have completed both the original *Get Buffed!*™ program, as well as this more advanced, second generation *Get Buffed!*™ II : Get More Buffed! program. Over and above any fantastic training effects you have achieved, I trust I have also significantly advanced your ability to make decisions about training - the what, when, how and why about training, recovering and eating.

The *Get Buffed!*™ range began with the original *Get Buffed!*™ book, and is now an extensive range of educational material for any person wanting to enhance their physique and physical capacity through strength training. All of these products are available at the *Get Buffed!*™ web site, www.getbuffed.net.

I want to thank you for trusting your training adaptations to the theories and methods I have shared through the *Get Buffed!*™ range. As you know, my goal has never been to teach you any one training method or belief. But rather, to teach you that they all have a place at some time in your career, and more importantly – that you have the power to make the decisions!

Not only do you have the power, you are the best positioned person to interpret the feedback from your training and recovery program. You are the only person with you all day and night long.

Enjoy the information and sample training programs provided in this book and other *Get Buffed!*™ products. Take a long-term view to your training. Maintain your health. And go and *Get Buffed!*™

Ian King

About The Author

Ian King was born and raised on an island in the Pacific. It was there he developed a passion for sport. In addition to being involved in many sports, he began his strength training career at the early age of seven years old.

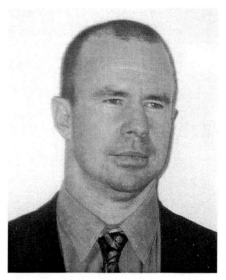

For the bulk of his adult life Ian has been committed improving the sporting success of elite athletes. His involvement with athletes in over 10 countries and over 20 sports has provided a rare and ideal opportunity to develop successful physical preparation methods applicable to the multi-year development of the athlete.

He has prepared athletes for every winter and summer Olympic Games since 1988, and every Commonwealth Games since 1984, as well as World Championships and World Cups in numerous sports. However he doesn't count the medals - he believes that credit should stay with the athlete.

Ian has taken the lessons he has learnt from training elite athletes over many years and applied them to training programs to benefit every person committed to developing their bodies through strength training. He is sharing the methods he developed from both his personal and professional experience. Ian belief's in training that training should be fun and rewarding, that training is for life, and that there is a little part in all of us that has a desire to *Get Buffed!*™

About The Get Buffed! ™ Product Range

Get Buffed!™ is range of strength training educational material by Ian King. Drawing from his extensive personal and professional experiences in strength training, Ian has created a collection of educational material to help you Get Buffed!™ Ian's goal is simple — to elevate the training results of everyone using strength training. The training methods being shared with you in the Get Buffed!™ range have been extremely well received. Why? Because they work!

The Get Buffed!™ Newsletter   Free subscription to readers of this book
The Get Buffed!™ Newsletter! is packed with TONS of invaluable information. We are covering tons of topics that will help and inspire you achieve your goals to use your time and efforts more effectively than ever before - to create a physique that is more than you could ever have imagined! Subscribe to this newsletter by emailing to newsletter@getbuffed.net with the words SUBSCRIBE GET BUFFED in the subject field.

Get Buffed!™ I – Ian King's Guide to Getting Bigger, Stronger & Leaner
$39.95 USD
Get Buffed!™ is not just 'another bodybuilding' book! It takes Ian's theories and methods of strength training and explains them for all who use strength training - so they can benefit from these methods to improve themselves and their quality of life. Not just a narrow approach for bodybuilders - but information that will boost the results of weight trainers, athletes, bodybuilders, power lifters, Olympic lifters and anyone else who want to optimize their time and efforts in the gym. Get Buffed!™ contains over 300 pages and well over 100,000 words - of down to earth, no-holds barred, how Ian recommends you should go about getting bigger, stronger and leaner. And Get Buffed!™ contains more than just information. It contains a fully blown 12-week program based on the popular 4 day split. Read Get Buffed!™ and immediately improve your training and the results!

Ian King's Guide To Control Drills $29.95 USD

This video has Ian King demonstrating, with the use of an athlete, his approach to control/stability training. Control drills, as Ian calls them, can be quite complex and challenging to describe their execution in the written word - especially to do them in the special and unique way that Ian has his athlete's doing them! Make sure you are executing the movements in the way Ian intended by using this video series in conjunction with the program from the *Get Buffed!*™ book!

Ian King's Guide To Abdominal Training $29.95 USD

This video has Ian King demonstrating, with the use of an athlete, his approach to abdominal training. Abdominal exercises can be quite complex and challenging to describe their execution in the written word - especially to do them in the special and unique way that Ian has his athlete's doing them! Make sure you are executing the movements in the way Ian intended by using this video series in conjunction with the program from the *Get Buffed!*™ book!

Ian King's Guide To Individual Stretching $39.95 USD

This video has Ian King demonstrating, with the use of an athlete, his approach to individual stretching. Flexibility exercises can be quite complex and challenging to describe their execution in the written word - especially to do them in the special and unique way that Ian has his athlete's doing them! Make sure you are executing the movements in the way Ian intended by using this video series in conjunction with the program from the *Get Buffed!*™ book!

Ian King's Guide To the Bench Press $39.95 USD

After watching this video tape you will know exactly what Ian would have you doing in the bench press if he was coaching you and why. This tape covers many variables relating to the bench press. Body position variables such as feet placement, knee angle, scapula awareness, and head position. Equipment variables such as how to select the bench, bar and plates, chalk and wrist straps. Management issues such as warm-up, stretching, warm-up sets, arousal and recovery. Safety issues such as spotters and protecting your lower back. This tape also touches briefly on the bench press variations - including the incline, decline and dumbbell variations. And the tape concludes with a special section dedicated to more advanced issues such as arching and smelling salts.

Ian King's Guide To the Squat $39.95 USD

The squat is known as 'the king' of strength training exercises, and for good reason - it is a fantastic lift! This tape discusses many variables of the squat and their ramifications on the training effect. Body position variables such as feet width and angle, knee and hip movement, trunk and pelvis angles, and head position. Equipment variables such as rack height, how to select the bar and plates, and wrist and knee straps. Management issues such as warm-up, stretching, warm-up sets, arousal and recovery. Safety issues such as chalk, spotters and knee sleeves. This tape touches briefly on the squat variations - including the front squat, the split and overhead squat, and the single leg squat variations. And the tape concludes with a special section dedicated to more advanced issues such as belts and wraps, smelling salts and lifting suits.

Ian King's Guide To the Deadlift $39.95 USD

The deadlift does not have the same high profile as it's close relative the squat. Perhaps the poor perception of this lift is based on the way many do it - using momentum and leverage instead of working the muscles. This tape covers many variables relating to the deadlift. Body position variables such as feet width and angle, knee and hip movement, trunk and pelvis angles, and head position. Equipment variables such as how to select the bar and plates, chalk and wrist straps. Management issues such as warm-up, stretching, warm-up sets, arousal and recovery. Safety issues such as spotters and protecting your back. This tape touches briefly on the deadlift variations - including the stiff legged deadlift, the clean and high pull, and the single leg deadlift variations. And the tape concludes with a special section dedicated to more advanced issues such as belts and smelling salts.

Get Buffed!™ Training Diary $44.95 USD

Simple strategies like goal setting, monitoring your progress and recording your training could increase your training results. Without this training tool, you could waste years pushing yourself and getting only a percentage of the results you might with recording your training! Use the Get Buffed!™ training diary, and you will not only enhance your training results, but you will keep a record of all your training that you did through your training career. The Get Buffed!™ Training Diary has chapters dedicated to the recording of the following : Goal Setting and Analysis, Program Design, Strength Training, Flexibility Training, Speed Training, Endurance Training, Nutrition Analysis and Recommendations, Physical Assessment Records, Recovery Notes, and Goal Setting and Analysis. Use the different recording sections in this Training Diary and you'll have the power to drive towards your training goals at record speeds. You'll get the maximum return from every minute, and drop of sweat, you invest in your training!

Get Buffed!™ Video Series $137 USD

This video has Ian King demonstrating all the exercises in this four day split, 12 week (4 stage) *Get Buffed!*™ program! So if you have done this program, or are doing, or plan to do it, and you want some expert coaching - it doesn't get any better than this! Make sure you are executing the movements in the way Ian intended by using this video series in conjunction with the program from the *Get Buffed!*™ book!

Get Buffed!™ Pack 1 (Ian Kings Guide to Individual Stretching, Abdominal & Control Drills) $87 USD

Receive the Ian King's Guide to Individual Stretching, Abdominal Training and Control Drills as a pack and receive a 13% discount compared to ordering them individually!

Get Buffed!™ Pack 2 (Ian Kings Guide to the Squat, Bench Press & Deadlift) $107.00 USD

Receive the Ian King's Guide to the Squat, Bench Press and Deadlift as a pack and receive a 11% discount!

Get Buffed!™ Pack 3 (Ian Kings Guide to Stretching, Control Drills, Abdominals, Squat, Bench Press and Deadlift) $187.00 USD

Receive all six of the 'Ian King's Guide' videos - Control Drills, Individual Stretching, Abdominal Training, The Squat, The Bench Press and The Deadlift – as a pack and receive a 15% discount compared to ordering them individually!

Get Buffed!™ Total Package $377 USD

The *Get Buffed!*™ *Total Package* is the most cost effective way to get the full range of Ian King's *Get Buffed!*™ material. The *Get Buffed!*™ range is aimed at the end user in strength training and bodybuilding/shaping - those who just want to know how to do it themselves! The *Get Buffed!*™ *Total Package* includes the above ten (10) products - a mix books and videotape. In all you get $481.55 USD worth of product for $377 USD, a saving 22%!

Ian King's "Killer Leg Exercises for Strength and Mass" $39.95 USD

Ian King's "Killer Leg Exercises for Strength and Mass" is jam-packed with special techniques that will keep your leg training fresh and muscles growing. This video covers all the exercises used in the 'Limping' program as posted on the T-mag web site (see the **Articles** section for easy access to these programs). This video is only available by ordering directly from http://www.biotest-online.com.

Faster, Higher, Stronger with Charlie Francis and Ian King Video $167.00 USD

This video is from a 1-day seminar presented by Charlie Francis and Ian King. This video is a lower-end production but contains rare and unique footage of this historic moment - the first time ever these two great coaches have come together in a seminar. Note that this video, unlike all of the above videos, is not a professionally produced video. It was shot on a domestic type digital camera. However it's rare footage, which is why we make it available. You will rarely see Charlie Francis on video, and to date this is the only video of Charlie Francis and Ian King in the same seminar.

Topics covered include: an overview of speed - definition and sub-qualities; energy systems as they relate to speed events; training intensities to develop these specific energy systems; the concept of the intensity specific continuum; the stretch-shortening cycle; periodization of speed; specificity vs. transfer in the area of speed, strength, endurance and flexibility; strength training as it specifically relates to speed performance; on injury prevention in speed sports; training program design; and recovery methods. Throughout the there are a number of question and answer session that covered diverse topics and of great value!

New product developments are continually being developed. To learn more, go to www.getbuffed.net or email us at info@getbuffed.net.

King Sports International
www.getbuffed.net
info@getbuffed.net
Ph +1-775-327-4550 Fax +1-240-465-4873
1135 Terminal Way, Suite 209, Reno NV 89502, USA